Fibromyalgia
B A S I C S

Good Health and Joy! Patti Chandler

Fibromyalgia
BASICS

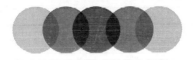

A Beginner's Guide

Pati Chandler

TATE PUBLISHING & *Enterprises*

Published by Tate Publishing & Enterprises, LLC
127 E. Trade Center Terrace | Mustang, Oklahoma 73064 USA
1.888.361.9473 | www.tatepublishing.com

Tate Publishing is committed to excellence in the publishing industry. The company reflects the philosophy established by the founders, based on Psalm 68:11,
"The Lord gave the word and great was the company of those who published it."

Book design copyright © 2011 by Tate Publishing, LLC. All rights reserved.
Cover design by Amber Gulilat
Interior design by Nathan Harmony

Published in the United States of America

ISBN: 978-1-61739-924-4
1. Health & Fitness / Reference
2. Health & Fitness / Pain Management
11.02.22

Dedication

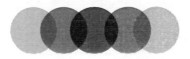

This book is dedicated to all those who live with this mysterious syndrome called fibromyalgia and to those who suspect they may have it, whether it appears by itself or along with any other chronic illness. As it haunts your days and nights, know that you are *not* alone.

Disclaimer

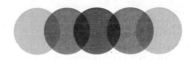

The information contained herein is not intended to diagnose or treat any illness, nor is it intended as a substitution for care from a professional. Please seek advice, diagnosis, medical treatment, and care from a trained health care practitioner.

Acknowledgments

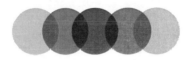

I want to thank Arlene Van Belle, Anita Cibelli, and Artie Estridge, my own personal "Triple A" club, without whose inspiration and encouragement this book would never have been written.

I thank Dr. Kumar Bhatt for his early diagnosis. I also thank him for his faith in me and in my writing endeavors.

A great big thank you to the Fibromyalgia Support Group in Mishawaka, Indiana, for sharing all their valuable support, input, inspiration, and encouragement.

I thank my family for their patience, understanding, good wishes, and their love.

Table of Contents

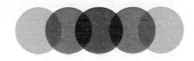

Foreword

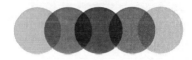

Imagine a poorly treated, significantly debilitating medical condition that millions suffer from, for which there is very little effective treatment. The medical establishment is unreceptive to recognizing it as a bona fide condition. Diagnosing it is clouded by the fact that there are no conclusive tests to verify its presence. What am I referring to? Depression, circa 1980.

The ensuing years have brought about a gradual recognition of this debilitating condition. Discovery of effective treatments for it has resulted in enormous numbers of people getting their lives back. And now a diagnosis of depression is well accepted by both patients and doctors alike as a very real and treatable condition.

Today, fibromyalgia is in the same situation that depression was initially. As the awareness of fibromyalgia increases, more and more people will recognize that this is the condition they themselves have and that there is hope for a better life.

This small book is one step in that direction. Its simple language and concise nature allow one to readily grasp the concepts involved in the physiology of this disease and, more importantly, the options in its treatment. Pati Chandler has crystallized her own experience of years of painful suffering coupled with painstaking research to give us this gem.

—Kumar Bhatt, DO
The Mishawaka Clinic
Mishawaka, Indiana

Introduction

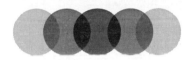

In the winter of 1998 I began exhibiting symptoms of fibromyalgia. Of course, I didn't know that then. I just knew that I hurt. Everywhere. All the time. Especially when I woke up in the morning. I was tired all the time; actually, exhausted would be more accurate. No matter how much sleep I was finally able to get, I never felt rested, much less refreshed. It seemed I felt even *more* tired when I woke up! I had lapses of memory and became easily confused. I seemed to be moving and acting in slow motion sometimes. There were times when I couldn't get my legs or arms to move the way I wanted them to; they felt as heavy as lead weights. Yet they seemed weak, as if the muscles were made of gelatin and I had no control over them.

More symptoms started showing up, one after the other after the other. One symptom seemed to have nothing to do with the other—they were all disconnected, like a hodge-podge of things gone wrong. Aside from feeling utter weakness and exhaustion, I felt confused and really scared. Depression set in. I felt like my body was suddenly falling apart and there was nothing I could do about it.

Other than one cold per year, I had never been sick and never needed a doctor for anything. But all this was more than I could take and certainly more than I wanted to deal with. I was getting progressively worse, and none of the symptoms were getting any better.

When I finally found the right doctor and was diagnosed, I came to understand that fibromyalgia was a chronic syndrome that would most likely last a lifetime. I knew I did not want to take prescriptions for the rest of my life, raising the doses regularly until … well, I didn't want to think about what my life would be like on painkiller prescriptions for next ten years, or twenty or thirty. I asked my doctor if there was anything natural I could take. Because he is an osteopath, he is open to such a request, thank heaven. He gave me the names of two supplements and two Web sites.

I began researching that very day. It was a long, slow process, given my mental "hiccups," as I called them, but the supplements began to help within three days. I started sleeping ... normally. What a concept! Some pain was still there, but it was not at all what it had been—at least I could think straight. I got online and went to complementary and alternative medical (CAM) Web sites such as The University of Maryland School of Medicine, The University of Michigan Pain and Fatigue Research Center, The National Institute of Health, The Mayo Clinic, and many more. I took copious notes. I trial and erred practically everything. It took me one full year, but I eventually found the right combination of stress management techniques, movements, foods, pacing, treatments, supplements, and of course avoidance of the specific factors that aggravated my symptoms. I had finally learned how to manage my symptoms. As a result, I have not found the need to visit that wonderful doctor for fibromyalgia symptoms since the year 2000. I see him now as a dear friend who literally saved my life—not to mention the *quality* of my life.

Recently, during a period of one week, no less than ten people came into my life that have been diagnosed with fibromyalgia—one in a wheelchair. Each recounted their tales. One woman said her doctor told her that fibromyalgia is a myth—a "catch-all diagnosis" for other doctors who couldn't find the "right" diagnosis. So he wrote her a prescription for each of her symptoms—eight in all, including an opioid for pain. Another woman told me that her doctor could find nothing wrong after all the expensive tests he'd ordered and so he could not, in good conscience, prescribe anything. She begged him for something to help her sleep, so he finally did write her a prescription for Ambien. Later he also wrote her a prescription for an antidepressant because she seemed so upset by the whole ordeal. Yet another woman said her doctor made an appointment for her with a psychiatrist because he could find nothing positive on any tests, leading him to believe it was probably an emotional thing.

As you can imagine, all these stories and others made my teeth grind in frustration.

I knew that there were many, *many* things that a person can do to help their symptoms, either in conjunction *with* medications or in place of them. I promptly gathered all my notes from back in 1998 and got to work making new notes—*lots* of them.

This book is the result of my accumulated research.

It is my hope that this book will help show you how to manage your symptoms by showing you some of the many options available, options you never knew you had.

It is time to bring your symptoms under *your* control. Fibromyalgia doesn't have to control you, not with all that is available for your choosing.

Fibromyalgia

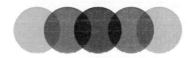

The word itself conjures up a multitude of feelings in the more than twelve million Americans who have fibromyalgia.[1] To those who don't have it, the word only brings a "what's that?" query. It is a rather new word to the English language, having been coined a little more than two decades ago. When broken down into its three parts (*fibro*, Latin for fibrous tissue; *myo*, Greek for muscle; and *algia*, Latin for pain), it is fairly self-explanatory. Simple.

Not so with the explanation of the condition, or syndrome. Because a syndrome, by definition, is a collection of symptoms, this is the most accurate term. So the condition is often called fibromyalgia syndrome, or FMS.

Fibromyalgia is considered an arthritis-related condition, which, according to the National Institute of Health, means it's a medical condition that impairs the joints and soft tissues and causes chronic pain.[2] It turns out to be much more than that, however, due to the multitude of symptoms that surround this condition.

Fibromyalgia is not a one-treatment-fits-all kind of a syndrome. Each person's fibromyalgia manifests somewhat differently, making it extremely difficult for physicians to treat. And though the symptoms are many and varied, they intertwine to "make up" the syndrome, with pain and fatigue the common denominator.

Symptoms

What are the symptoms? "Practically everything known to man" would be the answer given by a person with fibromyalgia. But pain is the symptom that tops the list and pretty much defines the entire subject. Muscular pain. Joint pain. Neck pain. Headache pain. Jaw and facial pain. Lower back pain. Upper arm pain. Wrist pain. Hip pain. Leg pain. Foot pain. Many or all of the above. In other words, think a severe case of the flu where everything hurts, the muscles and joints in the body don't work properly, and utter exhaustion rules the day.[3]

With a major flare-up, the pain in each of those places is severe and sharp. These flare-ups are generally brought on by some instigating factor, or aggravator, which amplifies the pain and/or other symptoms to acute levels. When the flare-up subsides, the pain is still there—it virtually never goes away because fibromyalgia is a chronic malady. This pain, however, is now in the form of constant and relentless aches all over. This pain is not as totally debilitating as the more extreme flare-up, but in its own way, it can be even more insidious. The constant dull aches and pains are so unmercifully persistent and constant that it's no wonder depression is a common symptom. It simply wears a body down. The Colorado River carving the Grand Canyon deeper and deeper comes to mind.

Pain is only the first symptom. The full list of symptoms is a legion. An individual may not have all the symptoms, but it is very common to have most of them. They include but are not limited to an all-consuming fatigue, numbness or tingling sensations in the hands and feet, sudden momentary electric-shock-like sensations in the hands and feet, irritable bowel syndrome, restless leg syndrome, dizziness, lowered resistance to infection, and chemical sensitivity, inhaled or ingested. Odors, food additives, or even some medications can initiate either allergy symptoms, like burning eyes and throat with runny nose, *or* body symptoms, like nausea, headache, dizziness, vomiting, and body pain.

There is a heightened sensitivity to touch, cold, heat, odors, noise, and bright lights, in addition to memory difficulties and confusion (sometimes called fibro fog), anxiety or panic attacks, abdominal pain with bloating and/or nausea, and moodiness. Some symptoms actually mimic other conditions, such as chronic fatigue syndrome, carpal tunnel syndrome, arthritis, even lupus, multiple sclerosis, and Alzheimer's.[4]

The most common symptom for all people with fibromyalgia is a total lack of deep, restful, restorative, stage four sleep. This is the period of sleep where the body repairs and replenishes itself, healing the multitudinous tiny tears in muscle tissue we all get during the day, when our body brings in oxygen to those areas that have become depleted during the day.[5] During every eight-hour night of sleep, those with FMS are constantly interrupted by bursts of awake-like brain activity prohibiting stage four sleep.

In other words, there is a malfunction at the most basic level—the level at which the body should be healing itself.[6] For those without FMS, it would be akin to just drifting off to sleep then jerking awake constantly, all night long … *every* night.

It's no wonder FMS sufferers wake up feeling like they have been dragged a mile down a railroad track. And they wake exhausted. Some sufferers have reported that getting out of bed in the morning involved crawling on hands and knees just to get to the bathroom. All-over body pain upon waking is a symptom all FMS sufferers endure.

The painful muscles are weak and don't move properly. The aching legs and ankles feel like lead weights are attached to them, and walking becomes a not-so simple task. Holding a cup of coffee must be done with two hands due to weak arms and wrists or tingly and numb hands and fingers.

The memory difficulties and confusion that are so prevalent with fibromyalgia sufferers are no less imposing.[7] The mind tends to wander in the middle of what you are saying or doing. If driving, for example, forgetting where you are going or even how to get home is a very scary proposition, and a panic attack can occur. But then a panic attack can also occur while standing at the kitchen sink doing the dishes.

Adding insult to injury, another symptom for some is weight gain, which usually adds to depression.[8] Clumsiness and spatial difficulties are not exactly morale boosters either.

With fibromyalgia, every day is different. From day to day, the frequency and location of pain and degree of the pain varies—from general body aches to severe and debilitating pain, along with any of the *other* added symptoms that decide to show up.[9]

The Cause

No one knows what causes fibromyalgia, although researchers have many theories. Some think that the lack of sleep may be a cause rather than a symptom. Another theory suggests changes in the muscle metabolism caused by decreased blood flow, and thereby low oxygen flow, to the muscles may be a cause.[10]

Experts have noted that fibromyalgia often manifests after an injury or trauma (particularly in the upper spinal region) or following a viral or bacterial infection, such as a severe case of bronchitis or the flu. In fact, it can manifest following, or along with, any incident that lowers the body's resistance. This is when its fighting forces are at its lowest ebb—this includes emotional trauma or severe stress as well.[11]

Most experts agree that it may be a central nervous system disorder, citing that the nervous system may be supersensitive in some way. Researchers have found elevated levels of a pain-producing nerve chemical, called substance P, in the spinal fluid of FMS sufferers, while at the same time finding too little of the neurotransmitter serotonin, which helps modulate pain perception, mood, sleep, and more. [12]

Others are looking deeper into the malfunctioning of the HPA axis, hypothalamus-pituitary-adrenal glands, which includes the thyroid and other hormones.[13]

All the above factors are known to exist in those with fibromyalgia, but whether they are the cause or not is another matter.

There have been studies leading some to believe that fibromyalgia is genetic and all that's required is a "trigger," like an auto accident, a severe bronchial infection, or a catastrophically stressful event. Some think it may be caused by a yet unknown virus or microbe of some kind. Some think it may be linked to Lyme disease in some way.[14] Theorizing and testing is still going on. But there is still no definitive cause that can be pointed to and declared, "That's what causes it." At least not yet.

Medical Help

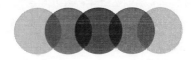

Fibromyalgia starts out as a mystery even unto the patient. In some cases many of these symptoms can show up all at once. But often it may seem like you are falling apart one symptom at a time, until there is such a collection of symptoms that you believe you have collected all the diseases of the twentieth century.

You may begin to experience wrist pain similar to carpal tunnel syndrome. The sides of your thighs or hips may begin to hurt or feel so weak it's physically difficult to lift your leg to go upstairs. Your upper arms may ache or feel so weak and shaky that you can't reach up in the cupboard for a glass. And you need two hands to hold that glass because your wrists and fingers are so numb and tingly that you can't even feel the glass in your hands. You may feel utterly weak and exhausted without having done anything to warrant it. You may begin to feel extremely forgetful or clumsy. You may wake up feeling more tired than when you went to bed and hurt all over as if you slept on cold concrete all night. You may suddenly begin to get headaches or allergies when you never had them before. You may find yourself using the bathroom much more often than usual. You may feel bloated and extremely uncomfortable, as if you've eaten a full course turkey dinner, when you've only had a small meal or even just a snack.

One after the other after the other, accumulating, compounding your feelings of "everything going wrong!" Yes, fear comes into play. It seems there can be no way to get back to normal when everything is falling apart.

See your doctor. You may even need to visit multiple doctors in a variety of specialties before finding out anything definitive. This alone is exhausting … and depressing. But stick with it. Finding the right doctor or health care practitioner *for you and your fibromyalgia symptoms* is extremely important and can greatly ease your stress. This is especially important because we know that stress is one of the main aggravators.

Diagnosis

Diagnosing fibromyalgia is a bit of a problem. This is because fibromyalgia doesn't show up in blood tests, on X-rays, on CT scans, or even on a standard MRI. When the FMS sufferer tells his or her doctor the list of symptoms—usually after weeks of feeling all-over pain, weakness, and utter exhaustion—the doctor will run a battery of tests to eliminate the usual suspects displaying these and all the rest of the symptoms. The doctor will test for hypothyroidism, multiple sclerosis, rheumatoid arthritis, lupus, and so on.[15] All the tests come up negative. Now this should be a good thing. And it is, sort of. At least these serious disorders have been eliminated. The problem lies in the criteria for the diagnosis.

The diagnosis of fibromyalgia requires only two conditions. The first is that the pain must have been consistent for at least three months. That alone does not sound hopeful. The second condition is that eleven of eighteen tender points should demonstrate pain when slight pressure is applied.[16] (See illustration.)

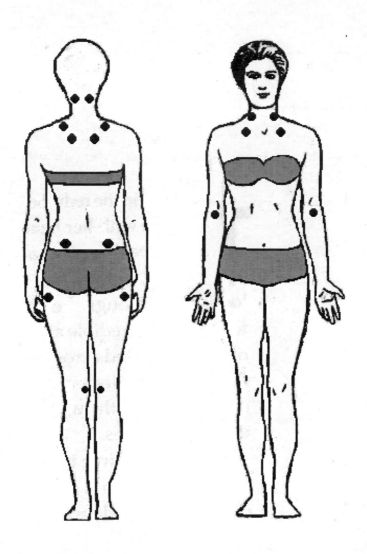

In a non-FMS sufferer there would be no pain at all when these points are pressured. But if fibromyalgia is the culprit, a slight pressure applied to these points will create a bone-deep, radiating, lasting pain at these sites. This is not an enjoyable procedure. But it is necessary for the proper diagnosis. In recent years, many general practitioners, rheumatologists, osteopaths, naturopaths, even chiropractors and acupuncturists have learned about this diagnostic method and can confirm whether you do indeed have fibromyalgia.

There is good news and bad news with a diagnosis of fibromyalgia. The good news is that fibromyalgia is not progressive or life threatening. The bad news is that it is chronic, that is, long-lasting.[17]

Okay. You have a diagnosis—a label. Now what? Knowledge is power. Educate yourself about the syndrome. Google it! Keyword it! Learn all you can through Web sites such as those listed in the chapter "Bountiful Resources," through books, articles, and so on. There is information everywhere now, and it's updated constantly. Medical testing goes on daily. And individual essays and books such as this are meant for all FMS sufferers in hopes that something that helps one may help others. Each FMS sufferer must learn what his or her medical options are, learn what aggravates the symptoms, and learn about self-care. Learn what you can do to manage your own health and well-being.

Physicians

In 1990 the American College of Rheumatology established the general classification guidelines for this syndrome, and they have subsequently done much of the research involved in its assessment. In fact, rheumatologists Richard H. Gracely, Frank Petzke, Julie M. Wolf, and Daniel J. Clauw from the University of Michigan Health System—Chronic Pain and Fatigue Research Center actually proved, via functional magnetic resonance imaging (fMRI), that fibromyalgia was a legitimate, painful, medical condition and *not* an imagined ailment as had been believed for many years.[18]

Family practitioners are learning more and more about this syndrome as more and more cases appear in their practice. But those who are the most successful at treating this complicated syndrome are those who practice integrative medicine. Integrative medical physicians are those who utilize the best of modern Western medicine in conjunction with the proven beneficial three-thousand-year-old traditional medicines and treatments.

Osteopathic physicians and a number of Western-trained medical physicians are finding that fibromyalgia responds best to a well-blended marriage of the two forms of medicine—this is integrating medicines and treatments. Naturopathic physicians are also known to be quite successful at treating fibromyalgia, combining a variety of successful treatments and techniques of their own.

But whether a family physician, a rheumatologist, an osteopath, a naturopath, or an integrative medical physician, almost everyone involved in the care and treatment of fibromyalgia, as well as those who suffer from the syndrome, agrees that the two most important treatments are for restorative, restful sleep and pain relief.

Sleep

Unfortunately, regular sleeping pills haven't proved helpful for FMS sufferers because they don't address stage four sleep. However, there are several prescription medications that help. A low dosage tricyclic antidepressant, such as amitriptyline, e.g. Elavil, or a muscle relaxant, such as cyclobenzaprine, e.g. Flexeril, has been shown to help get that restorative, healing sleep. Also, a different type of antidepressant called a selective serotonin and norepinephrine reuptake inhibitor (SNRI) has been effective.[19]

Even though the tricyclic antidepressants and the SNRIs are prescribed for FMS sufferers in a fraction of the dose given for clinical depression, these and all medications are not meant to be used *ad infinitum*. Because fibromyalgia is a chronic syndrome, it may be necessary over a lengthy period of time to adjust dosages of these medications and/or alternate medications in order to avert dependence or adaptation.

Some physicians may recommend an over-the-counter antidepressant called Sam-e, short for S-adenosylmethionine.[20] In Europe, Sam-e is a prescription medication, and physicians there have prescribed it for depression, chronic fatigue syndrome, and fibromyalgia for many years. See "Herbs and Supplements" for further description.

> Note: Before taking any supplements, check with your health care provider (HCP). Always

tell your HCP of any medications or supplements you are currently taking.

Pain Relief

What is the first thing recommended by health care practitioners (HCPs) for relief of fibromyalgia pain? Exercise. That's right—exercise. It sounds all too cruel to tell a person suffering the exhaustion and muscular and joint pains of fibromyalgia that he or she should exercise. But, believe it or not, the reasoning is sound.

It's because physical exercise releases the body's own natural pain-relieving chemicals called endorphins, which loosely translated means "the body's natural morphine." Exercise has been *proven* to alleviate much of the pain of fibromyalgia.[21]

Pain management programs referred by your HCP or local medical facility can be of tremendous help. The physical therapists at these pain management facilities understand physical pain and work with you. We're not talking Tae Bo or jumping jacks here. These are exercises for pain management. Gentle, slow, five-minute "workouts" of low or no-impact stretches are all that's required at first to get those endorphins charged up again. The physical therapist will guide and direct movements that have been choreographed especially for you and your needs. Once you've learned the movements, you can then do them at home anytime for pain relief.

Start low and go slow. Add a minute or two each week to your regimen. The relief after each session is truly a blessing.

In severe cases of fibromyalgia, especially during a major flare-up, trigger point injections of an analgesic or cortisone medication given directly at the tender point sites have proven to be helpful in relieving soft tissue pain and breaking up severe muscle spasms.[22]

But for the relentless and constant day-to-day pain, there is really very little that the medical community can do. Normal pain relievers, such as aspirin, acetaminophen, nonsteroidal anti-inflammatory drugs (NSAIDS)—such as ibuprofen, naproxyn, or Aleve— or even Cox II inhibitors, such as Celebrex, have not proven to be very effective for the pain of fibromyalgia. Narcotic pain relievers and corticosteroids, such as prednisone, haven't been shown to be very effective for fibromyalgia pain either, especially for the long haul.

However, in June of 2007, the FDA approved the use of an anticonvulsant named Lyrica (Pfizer

Incorporated) for use in the treatment of fibromyalgia. And in June of 2008, Cymbalta (Eli Lilly and Company) was approved by the FDA for treating fibromyalgia—this is an antidepressant and SNRI (serotonin and norepinephrine reuptake inhibitor) combination. Then in January of 2009, the FDA approved a third drug, also an antidepressant and SNRI, called Savella (Forrest Pharmaceuticals) for treating fibromyalgia.[23]

Be aware, however, that because chemical sensitivity is one of the symptoms that many FMS sufferers endure, some chemical treatments may not be handled well by a fibromyalgic body and may even act in reverse, amplifying symptoms.

If your HCP prescribes any of these medications, please be certain to let him or her know immediately if side effects are experienced, if symptoms become worse, or if you begin experiencing even more symptoms than before.

Your health care provider may also have recommendations as to activities or conditions to avoid. These would be called aggravators. And there are foods which can aggravate pain and/or other symptoms. These are called edible aggravators.

Aggravators

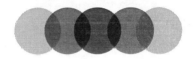

 Identifying activities, conditions, even *things* that aggravate this syndrome is essential to managing fibromyalgia. You must become a detective and find out for yourself what your specific aggravators are. You may find it helpful to write down the day and time when a flare-up occurs. Then jot down what you did, what you ate, what was going on when it happened, or even the day *before* it happened.

This will help you find out what some of your personal aggravators are. Suggested aggravators are listed below and in the following chapter, but you may find your own not listed here. Keeping a journal of this sort, whether it is in the form of an actual written journal, an iPod, a Blackberry, or whatever, also helps you remember what to tell your HCP what you were feeling when you began to hurt, how long, and so on.

The list of various and potential aggravators is long and diverse, but thirteen of the most common aggravators are listed here; then each is explored in more detail with suggestions for how to minimize them. The most common edible aggravators are explored in the following chapter.

List of Aggravators

1. Lack of restorative sleep

2. Intense pain upon waking

3. Lack of exercise

4. Too much exercise

5. Stress (at home and/or work)

6. Hormonal fluctuations (menses or menopause)

7. Changes in weather

8. Cold and drafty conditions (winter *and* summer air-conditioning)

9. Erratic daily schedule (at home and/or work)

10. Repetitive movements (at home and/or work)

11. Sitting or standing for a lengthy period of time

12. Sitting on soft or overstuffed furniture

13. Sleeping on a hard or extra firm mattress

Minimizing these and any other aggravators the FMS sufferer may discover in his or her own specific case is a big step toward managing fibromyalgia pain.

Minimizing Thirteen Aggravators

1. Lack of Restorative Sleep

Start with the obvious. Talk to your doctor. It is helpful, immediately after diagnosis, to hit the sleep issue with the big guns—with the prescription medications of Elavil or Flexeril for example. With normal sleep, which *includes* the healing stage four sleep, the body can begin to repair itself and bring in the oxygen it needs on a daily basis. After a couple of months, when the body is once again familiar with normal sleep, you may consider switching to a natural supplement, like 5-HTP or melatonin (see "Herbs and Supplements"), and phase off prescriptions altogether.

Prescriptions and supplements aren't the only way to get sleep, though. You need to do your part too. This includes some of the age-old commonsense factors, such as:

- Avoid caffeine and alcohol in the afternoon and evening. This includes soft drinks, chocolate, and some medications.

- Avoid spicy foods or drinking water before bed. Heartburn and/or trips to the bathroom don't allow for a peaceful night's sleep.

- On the other hand, a glass of warm milk or a cup of chamomile tea can be helpful to many.

- Avoid exercising at least three hours before bedtime. Although exercise creates endorphins for helping pain, it is also stimulating and can keep you awake.

- Give yourself time to wind down before bed. Avoid working around the house or on the computer or any mentally taxing chores before bed.

- Take a soothing bath, listen to relaxing music, or read a couple of chapters of a soothing novel (no suspense or horror novels, please). Relax your body as well as your mind before going to bed.

- Go to bed at approximately the same time every night. Regularity of a schedule is very important. Your body needs to understand that this time of night is for sleep.

- Keep the sleeping room for sleep. A television, computer, telephone, and so on in the bedroom are there to keep you alert. (This includes your cell phone.) A dark, cool, *quiet* atmosphere is much more conducive to sleep.

- Deep breathing exercises, relaxation techniques, and visualization exercises are very helpful.

2. Intense Pain upon Waking

For fibromyalgia sufferers, the hardest part of the day is getting out of bed after lying still for hours at a time. Remaining in one position for any length of time is not in the best interest of a painful fibromyalgic body.[24]

Upon waking in the morning, try the toe and ankle exercise.

Toe and Ankle Exercise

Before you get out of bed, turn to lie on your back. With feet together (as if your big toes were tied together), heels resting on the bed, use your ankles to *slowly* draw large circles with your big toes—first clockwise four times then counterclockwise four times. Rest.

Then scrunch the toes on your left foot as if grabbing something. Hold for a count of four. Relax your toes. Then scrunch the toes on your right foot. Hold for a count of four. Relax your toes. Repeat four times with each foot. Rest.

Now point your left foot toward the end of the bed while pointing your right foot toward your forehead. Hold for a count of four.

Reverse positions, pointing your right foot toward the end of the bed, your left toward your forehead. Hold for a count of four. Repeat four times with each foot. Rest.

Now turn on your side for a few minutes (either side will do) and lay in a comfortable fetal position with your pelvis tipped forward but relaxed. Then slowly, gently, get out of bed. The pain will be *much* less severe upon rising. Guaranteed.

These exercises get the blood flowing throughout your body. As if starting a car on a cold winter morning, it gets the fluids flowing through your engine before putting it in gear.

The toe and ankle exercises are excellent for anyone, with or without fibromyalgia, who sits at a desk or in a car, on a train or a plane for long periods. They get the blood flowing in the lower extremities and help in breaking up any toxins that settle there over a lengthy period of time. These exercises are also extremely important for anyone at risk for DVT, deep vein thrombosis.

3. Lack of Exercise

Lack of movement creates pain in a fibromyalgic body.[25] Exercise, in fibromyalgic terms, however, does *not* mean strength training, weight lifting, or jogging. Walking from the front of the house to the back of the house can constitute exercise for a person with fibromyalgia. Walking to the end of the block and back is exercise. Walking up a flight of stairs…you get the idea. This may not seem like much to non-FMS sufferers, but for someone with fibromyalgia, these little trips can be daunting at times. However, they *are* examples of exercise. Anyone who suffers from fibromyalgia *must* move—then rest, then move.[26] We call it exercise for lack of a better term. "Moving" is more accurate.

Do what you can, but *do*. Regularly. Shrug your shoulders, gently shake your hands, "march" your arms, or do the toe and ankle exercises. The object here is to get the blood flowing to your muscles, taking the healing oxygen and nutrients with it.

When you're feeling strong enough, go to the library and check out DVDs (or VHS tapes) such as *Tai Chi For Arthritis*, *Stretching for Seniors* (no matter what your age), or similar videos that demonstrate minimal *gentle* exercise. See the suggested list in the chapter "Bountiful Resources."

At home you can try each at your own pace. Just watching the slow, gentle, rhythmic movements of tai chi is relaxing and soothing. The benefits of doing these exercises and stretches are a testament unto themselves in the minimizing of fibromyalgia pain. When you find a video that works well for you, invest in a copy of it for your own personal library. Doing these exercises or stretches with a group is ideal, but doing it with a group on a video is the next best thing.

The very best thing about these videos is that it is easy to pace yourself. You can stop the DVD every five minutes if you want, sit down and rest any time you want, and skip over anything you want. You can make up your own exercise regimen using one movement from one DVD, two from another, and so on. There is no one there to tell you otherwise.

Tip: One very important fact of *any* exercise regimen is to remember that what you do on the right side you must do equally on the left. This is especially true for a fibromyalgic body. All four quadrants must get the benefit of the blood and oxygen flowing through those muscles—left and right above the waist, and left and right below the waist. Balance is the key.

A regular exercise routine of five minutes a day (or a couple of times a day), then expanding on it next week to six or seven minutes a day and so on—up to fifteen or twenty minutes a day in a month or two if you can—will bring untold relief from the most severe pain. Remember, start low and go slow.

Create a habit for health. Five or ten minutes (or more) every morning start the day off with those endorphins working *for* you. Getting into the habit of an exercise regimen can be the very best thing you can do for yourself. You will definitely feel better, and you'll find it is extremely meditative and calming. If you're having a painful day, do a two-minute exercise. But do it.

Mornings are ideal for exercising, but early afternoon is good for a pick-me-up during a taxing day. As stated earlier, however, don't do these energizing exercises two or three hours before bed, as they are not conducive to sleep.

4. Too Much Exercise

Too much exercise exacerbates fibromyalgic pain; that's obvious to anyone with fibromyalgia. But how much is too much? This becomes self-evident when it occurs. Learn your limitations. It's true; these limitations may adjust as these aggravators get more under control, but in the meantime, accept that you simply cannot do what you did before fibromyalgia. Your body is telling you that change is needed. Listen to it.

Pace yourself realistically for the condition you're in. Just because you feel pretty good today doesn't mean that you should go all out and get everything done that's been piling up for the past week. Doing so often causes your body to retaliate for the next two or even *three* days, in the form of a nasty flare![27] Pacing includes the *good* days too ... whenever you have them. Think ahead. Plan ahead. Pace yourself.

5. Stress

It's now common knowledge how much damage stress can do to a body, ranging from ulcers to a heart attack and all kinds of maladies in between, including depression. But illness itself is stressful to a body—

especially when it's been three or more months of the exhaustion, pain, and confusion of fibromyalgia. And now it seems that all those little things at home and work that were never stressful before have suddenly become disproportionately stressful. They may seem intolerable, even insurmountable.

Those with fibromyalgia *must* make the time to *de*-stress. [28] It's as simple as ABC. A is for air, B is for bye, and C is for count.

A. Learn to breathe. Close your eyes and take deep belly breaths. Breathe in through your nose, expanding your belly like a balloon, for a slow count of four. Hold it for a count of four. Then, through pursed lips, release your breath, pushing all the air out of your belly, to a slow count of four. Hold it for a count of four. Repeat as often as you wish. In with the good air, out with the bad.

B. Detach yourself. Physically. Temporarily set the issue aside. Go into the bathroom. Lock the door. Toss a towel onto the floor and take off your socks and shoes. Sit down on the toilet seat and grab the towel with your toes, alternating the right foot and the left. Breathe. *Note: When you lock yourself in the bathroom stall at work, there may be no towel, so grab your socks with your toes.*

C. Count. While in the bathroom (or stall), close your eyes, breathe, and count the big, white, puffy cumulous clouds drifting overhead. In your mind's eye, notice their shapes as they drift by—the irregular edges. Feel the puff of wind on your cheek as it pushes the cloud along and the next one drifts into view. Become aware of the stark white color of the cloud against the bright blue of the sky. Or count M&Ms. Visualize a huge pile of one million M&Ms. Mentally slide one off to the side, noticing its smooth, round texture and color as it easily slides over. Listen to the sound it makes as it slides. Mentally pull out another and slide it over, then another and another. Or count sheep or anything that has *nothing* to do with what is on the other side of that locked door.

These are called visualization techniques and can be very helpful in calming and *de*-stressing the body. The toe grips keep the muscles moving (many muscles, if you'll notice); the deep breathing oxygenates the blood and muscles; the visualization calms the stress chemicals. All three help bring the body back into balance. The moving center, the intellectual center, and the emotional center all come into balance. Make it a new habit. It will do the body good.

6. Hormonal Fluctuations

Medical assistance may be required here. Dr. Jacob Teitelbaum, author and leading authority on chronic fatigue syndrome and fibromyalgia, uses the acronym SHIN to address the treatment of the pain and fatigue of fibromyalgia. S is for sleep, H is for hormone balance, I is for infection control, and N is for nutritional support.

"The important thing," Dr. Teitelbaum says, "is that all four should be implemented in concert with one another for maximum therapeutic effect."[29]

In fact, hormonal fluctuations are often right smack in the middle of all the other FMS symptoms.

Whether PMS, peri-menopause, or post-menopause, when hormones begin hiccupping around in your body in such erratic fashion, fibromyalgia symptoms are nearly impossible to manage. It's all connected, you see.

Addressing the hormone factor is a *must* for managing fibromyalgia symptoms. Talk to your HCP or your endocrinologist. Again, if chemical sensitivity is a factor for you, it is helpful to use natural hormonal assistance. The previously mentioned ABC technique can be helpful here too.

7. Changes in Weather

There's not much one can do about the weather, unfortunately, but the FMS sufferer can prepare for it. Know what's coming in order to dress and act accordingly. In hot and humid weather, be especially careful not to overdo in the heat of the day. Excess perspiration depletes your store of electrolytes—magnesium, potassium, and calcium specifically—which can be most aggravating to those with fibromyalgia. This can definitely lead to muscle aches and weakness. Any outside activities, such as walking or gardening, are best done in the cooler early morning or late afternoon or dusk hours. Air-conditioning is a wonderful invention, but precautions may be needed. (See number eight.)

In cold and wet weather err on the side of too much clothing. Layers can always be taken off. In winter it helps to wear a hood attached to the coat instead of a hat with a coat. And zip up to your chin. The hood and high neck keep the cold wind off the back of the neck, front of the neck, and clavicle areas where tender points can be affected. When the muscles around these tender points suddenly contract or seize up due to the cold, pain/and or muscle spasms over the whole neck and shoulder area can take over. Don't get caught without the ability to cover up.

8. Cold and Drafty Conditions

Don't get caught without the ability to cover up. That is an intentional duplication. The importance of this cannot be stressed enough. A cold draft to the neck, shoulders, arms, and hips can cause cramps and pain to increase in intensity. In the summertime be sure to have a long-sleeved shirt handy. Keep one in the car in case it's needed to keep the chill of air-conditioning off those sensitive areas. All fabric stores have remnants where you can purchase a piece of fleece. Even a small eighteen-inch by sixty-inch remnant piece makes a great shoulder wrap in any weather. It also covers your neck from any drafts, and it's handy to lay over your cold feet or hands.

9. Erratic Daily Schedule

Home or work schedules that require waking, eating, and going to bed at different times every day can wreak havoc with fibromyalgia.[30] It is extremely important to wake, exercise, eat, work, and go to bed at the same general times every day. A regular routine enables the endorphins from exercise and work to be released at regular intervals. Medications and supplements should be taken daily at regular times. Irregular and constantly changing patterns in exercise, work, sleep, etc., prevent the medications, endorphins, the sleep cycle, and all the rest from working together efficiently to help ease the pain of fibromyalgia.

10. Repetitive Movements

Computer work, factory work, and even vacuuming require repetitive movements and create pain for a fibromyalgic body.[31] Shift positions every twenty minutes or so. Do something different—change hands, move your body in a different way. If allowed to continually do any one thing for a half hour or more, it becomes increasingly difficult to continue that motion. Movement and function may become erratic, not to mention extremely painful.

11. Sitting or Standing for a Lengthy Period of Time

Again, shift positions every twenty minutes or so. If sitting, stand up and walk around for several minutes.[32] If standing, walk or sit down for a several minutes. If walking, sit down or stand still for several minutes (and breathe). Shifting positions every twenty minutes acts like exercise in that the body feels much better *after* the movement. The longer one stays in a single position, the more difficult it is to move into another position. This may be one reason the body wakes up in so much pain in the morning. Refer to the toe and ankle exercises.

12. Sitting on Soft or Overstuffed Furniture

This posture bends the body into angles that apply pressure to those sensitive tender points, especially the lower back and hip areas, as well as the neck and shoulders. Ergonomically contoured, molded chairs can also be quite painful to the lower back and hip area. A flat-seated, straight-backed chair, believe it or not, is really quite comfortable for those with fibromyalgia. Good posture while sitting or standing keeps pressure *off* the tender points, easing pain and aiding function. The very best of all chairs is a flat-seated, straight-backed glider or rocking chair, with or without cushions. This allows the option of movement—always a good thing for a fibromyalgic body. These types of chairs actually aid circulation, getting the needed oxygen to muscles.

13. Sleeping on a Hard or Extra Firm Mattress

In the past we've been told that to get a good night's sleep it is necessary to have a good firm mattress. Not so for anyone with fibromyalgia. A firm mattress can actually apply pressure to some of those very painful tender points, the lower back and hip areas particularly. Adding a two or three-inch foam pad or a pillow-top pad to the existing mattress can help reduce this aggravator. Investing in a good air mattress where the softness can be adjusted is quite helpful for some, while the popular therapeutic foam mattresses have been helpful for others. Test before you buy. Your health and well-being is at stake here.

The Edible Aggravators

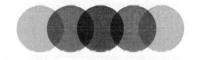

These are the aggravators that often go unnoticed. After all, you've been eating all your life; why all of a sudden would food of any kind be aggravating your symptoms? They never bothered you before. Therein lies the rub. Your body is different now. That difference often includes changes in your body's chemistry and its reaction to specific foods, especially those foods that contain excitotoxins and certain alkaloids, like aspartame, MSG, and nightshades. [33]

1. The Elimination Test

The best way to find out if your body is now sensitive to specific foods is to do an elimination test for each suspected food. To see if aspartame, for example, is an aggravating factor for you, you would perform an elimination test in the following manner: eliminate all foods and drinks that contain aspartame for a week to ten days—long enough to flush it out of your system. Then begin using those foods and drinks again. If a flare-up occurs in a day or two—sometimes two or three *hours* will tell—stop using the aspartame again and see if the flare-up subsides. If it does, count aspartame as an aggravator for you. Keep in mind that most sugar-free items, as well as some multivitamins and medicines, contain aspartame. Always check the labels.

2. Some Foods That Are Suspect

Aspartame (or any chemical sweetener), MSG, spicy foods, fried foods, excess sugar (or concentrated sugar, like high fructose corn syrup), and nightshades—a family of foods containing nerve-irritating alkaloids—have all been shown to aggravate painful symptoms in many people with fibromyalgia and in those with arthritis as well. Gluten and/or lactose intolerance are two more unsavory symptoms that appear in many with FMS.

Excess Sugar

According to Don Colbert, M.D., author of *The Seven Pillars of Health* (Siloam 2007), "Sugar in its natural state is always combined with fiber [e.g. fruits] to prevent sugar spikes and excessive release of insulin … but man has separated the fruit [sugars] from the fiber and created addictive foods."[34]

The more sugar you eat, the more you want. This is because sugar releases opioid-type chemicals in the brain that stimulate the desire for more sweets!

Excess sugar suppresses the immune system; it makes your blood more acidic; it greatly upsets the mineral balance within your cells; it increases free radicals within your body; it feeds yeast growth infections; it interferes with and creates imbalances in hormones. In fact, Nancy Appleton, Ph.D., author of *Lick The Sugar Habit* (Avery 1988), has listed—complete with medical resources—no less than 146 reasons why sugar is ruining your health![35]

Performing the elimination test with sugar, sugary foods, and foods with high fructose corn syrup can be quite enlightening. Hint: This pretty much covers everything in a box, package, can, or bottle in the grocery store!

Natural Sweeteners

If artificial sweeteners are an aggravator for you and you want to cut back on the real thing, consider using Stevia or Just Like Sugar—these are two all-natural, zero-calorie, zero-carb, zero-chemical sweeteners.

Stevia is made from the leaves of the stevia plant and is known to contain many vitamins, minerals, and antioxidants. It is 200–300 times sweeter than sugar and has a slight licorice aftertaste. Stevia, sold under several brand names, is available at most grocery and health food stores.

Just Like Sugar is made from chicory root, calcium, vitamin C, and orange peel. All four of these ingredients make it a fiber, a prebiotic, antioxidant, and more. The taste is exactly the same as sugar, in equal portions to cane sugar, and it has no aftertaste. It's available at Amazon.com and www.justlikesugarinc.com.

Both are real, live, natural, *healthful* sweeteners with zero calories! What more could you ask from a sweetener?

Nightshades

Do the elimination test with the nightshades, eliminating all white potatoes, tomatoes, bell peppers, chili peppers, and eggplants for a week to ten days. Chances are quite good that much of your pain can be greatly relieved. Then reintroduce them, one each week.

Nightshades contain certain alkaloids that can cause irritation and inflammation to nerve endings and joints in sensitive people, especially if consumed in large quantities. These alkaloids are accumulative, so eating all these delicious veggies at one time can literally make your body scream at you!

You may not have to give up all these delicious, antioxidant, and nutrition-rich vegetables, though. Most people who are sensitive to these alkaloids may do quite well by eating only one nightshade per meal or per day without any major symptoms showing up to spoil their day. Never combining two or more at any one meal may be just the ticket!

Caffeine

Caffeine can be an aggravating factor for some, coffee particularly. Try the elimination test. Some may do quite well by cutting back to one or two cups of coffee per day. You can also try drinking half hot water and half coffee, effectively diluting it enough to cause minimal effect.

The caffeine in tea, particularly green tea, is different because of its beneficial substance, L-Theanine, which nearly cancels out any jittery effect of caffeine.[36] In fact, L-Theanine is used in several over-the-counter sleep aids. And tea is full of antioxidants—always a good thing. Most herbal tea is naturally caffeine free.

Soft Drinks

The elimination test here will have startling results because of the long-term nature of the damage caused by these innocent-looking beverages. But whether they are diet or regular, soft drinks can *and do* create chronic pain and increase existing pain. Not just due to the sugar or aspartame, either of which can cause pain, but even more because of the phosphates. Phosphates bind with minerals in your body and literally steal calcium and magnesium from your muscle tissue and bones, causing pain and softening bones.[37] Over the course of years and years ... well, you can see where this could create problems like osteoporosis, arthritis, muscle weakness, etc.

Gluten, Lactose, and/or Yeast

Gluten: Wheat, barley, and rye have a complex protein that is difficult for many people to digest. (Oats may or may not be in this category.) If you are low in the proper enzymes, as in the case of someone who has gluten sensitivity or the more serious celiac disease, this not-so-innocent little protein can cause a world of problems, not just of the intestinal kind, but many other symptoms as well.[38]

Probiotics, such as those found in yogurt, are most important in helping to rebuild the intestine and promote healing from any damage done by gluten sensitivities. If milk products are an issue, probiotics, especially acidophilus, are also available in supplement form at health food stores and drugstores.

Lactose: Not only does milk contain a little protein molecule called *casein* that has the potential to wreak havoc; it also contains a well-known irritator called lactose. If you are lacking the enzyme lactase, as is a full 75 percent of the population of the world, you will find lactose difficult to digest and process, creating gastrointestinal issues, such as bloating, cramping, diarrhea, gas, etc. Lactose, of course, is found in milk and milk products. Many people without this enzyme can handle small amounts of milk products like cheese, yogurt, etc., without too many problems. If your sensitivity is mild, you can find the enzyme lactase as a supplement in health food stores and most drugstores to allow you to drink milk comfortably.[39]

Yeast: Jacob Teitelbaum, M.D., explains in his book *From Fatigued to Fantastic* (2007, Penguin Group) that yeast is a normal member of the body's "zoo." But when it overgrows its welcome and literally overruns the other members in the zoo, it causes major infection-type problems. This is actually more a product of a lowered immune system. And certain foods, like sugar and yeast-containing foods, feed this yeast so it can grow out of hand in a hurry, creating a myriad of unkind symptoms.[40]

Although not necessarily typical symptoms of fibromyalgia, gluten and/or lactose intolerance, as well as yeast overgrowth problems, are factors to be aware of and consider being tested for. See your HCP for a proper diagnosis.

You can do your own preliminary elimination test, but be aware that gluten and lactose are found in nearly every boxed, packaged, canned, and frozen food or drink in the grocery store, as well as supplements, over-the-counter medications, and prescriptions. So you'll need to learn how to find them. There are many Web sites with lists of gluten and lactose-containing foods, such as www.glutenfreeworks.com and www.foodintol.com. You can also Google "gluten sensitivity" and/or "lactose intolerance."

3. Essential Fatty Acids: the Extreme Ratio of Omega 6 to Omega 3

Omega 6 fatty acid has been inadvertently put in the position of being an aggravator. Actually, the inappropriate *ratio* of Omega 6 to Omega 3 has become the aggravator. These essential fatty acids *are* essential, and because our body doesn't produce them, we must get them through our diet. The problem is the ratio of the two *should* be two, or one to one. But according to the National Institute of Health (NIH), our Western diet has put it way out of balance at sixteen or twenty-five to one—far in favor of the inflammatory Omega 6.[41] (See "Then and Now.")

Inflammatories

This excess of Omega 6 fatty acids *increases* inflammation, blood clotting, water retention, and cell proliferation. It raises blood pressure, has a negative impact on the body's immune system, and may contribute to coronary heart disease, arrhythmia, obesity, depression, and some forms of cancer.

Anti-inflammatories

Omega 3 EPA-DHA, on the other hand, *decrease*s inflammation and aids in bringing down blood pressure and blood clotting, thereby reducing the risk of cardiovascular disease (CVD). Omega 3 EPA-DHA helps regulate arrhythmia, helps relieve water retention, lessens joint pain, and bolsters the immune system. It has also been shown to help alleviate anxiety, depression, and attention deficit disorder. Testing is still being done, and more and more benefits are being found when the ratio of Omega 6 and Omega 3 is closer to one to one.[42]

it or neutralized it by the processing. Omega 6 was and *is* practically indestructible.

The current high ratio between the two fatty acids (way too much Omega 6 and not enough Omega 3) leads to elevated proinflammatory cytokines, which has ultimately created an inflammation epidemic and enhanced the risk of numerous inflammatory diseases, such as osteoporosis, arthritis, type 2 diabetes, coronary heart disease, Alzheimer's, and many types of cancer.[44]

Everyone could benefit from adding Omega 3 EPA-DHA to their diets to help keep these chronic and inflammatory conditions at bay.

There is a little hitch in obtaining this beneficial fatty acid, however. Omega 3, containing the all-important EPAs and DHAs, is best obtained through eating dark meat fish like salmon, sardines, swordfish, herring, mackerel, and tuna. But eating two or three servings of these fish per week may be prohibitive. Also, according to the FDA, this amount may not be recommended due to possible mercury and PCB content that may be present in these fish.[45]

A good, high quality supplement of Omega 3 fatty acids (fish oil), containing the EPAs and DHAs the body needs, seems to be in order here. Fortunately, even the best quality Omega 3 supplements, usually from the Netherlands and the North Atlantic Ocean, are not expensive. And since the benefits of Omega 3 have been proven in test after test, study after study, it is well worth the investment to help alleviate one possible aggravator.

Omega 3 (and Omega 6) is found in walnuts, soy nuts, and flaxseed, as well as their oils. But, once again, if the oils are processed or the seeds are heated when used (or the walnuts cooked, as in baked cookies), the Omega 3 is neutralized, and you are left with only the Omega 6 fatty acid, adding to an already overabundance of Omega 6 in your body.

Jane Oelke, N.D., Ph.D., describes the role of essential fatty acids as helping to make the cell walls flexible and fluid, thereby contributing to the effective transfer of nutrients and oxygen into each cell.

In her book *Natural Choices For Fibromyalgia* (Natural Choices, 2001), she states, "The one supplement that has made the most difference [in treating fibromyalgia] is the use of essential fatty acids in the diet. If nutrients can't get into the cells, the body will never be healthy."[46]

So what is the ideal dosage of this important essential fatty acid? In nearly all of the thousands of studies and tests done by NIH, university medical schools, and medical centers, not to mention the many independent studies, the dosage commonly used is 1,000 mg–1,500 mg of EPA-DHA per day (1 gram–1.5 grams).[47] The EPA-DHA is what does the work, *not* the overall capsule of fish oil. Always check the label. Each capsule of 1,000 mg of fish oil contains a smaller amount EPA-DHA, 300 mg + 200 mg, for example. So if the total EPA-DHA per capsule is 500 mg, then two or three capsules per day will provide the recommended 1,000 mg–1,500 mg of EPA-DHA.

> Note: Before taking any supplements, check with your health care provider (HCP). Always tell your HCP of any medications or supplements you are currently taking.

Complementary Options

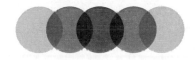

Complementary and alternative medicine (CAM) encompasses a whole range of treatments and modalities for easing pain, stress, balance, energy, and even your outlook on life. The options listed in this chapter cover only a few of the most well known, but there are many more. For a much more comprehensive list of CAM therapies, see Burton Goldberg's book *Alternative Medicine—The Definitive Guide* (Celestial Arts 2002) or go to www.healthy.net or www.umm.edu/altmed.

Support

Although not actually an alternative therapy, most people with fibromyalgia find a support group to be an extremely helpful therapy. A local fibromyalgia support group can be immensely supportive, especially when it's so hard to explain this syndrome to family, friends, and coworkers, not to mention the boss.

To find a support group, check newspapers, libraries, health food stores, your HCP's office, medical facilities, the YMCA, and anywhere else you can think of. If you can't find a fibromyalgia support group, try an arthritis support group. But make the effort. It can make a world of difference.

You can also find a group online at many of the fibromyalgia sites. And most of them even have newsletters where you can find out the latest news on research. Helpful sites are www.fibroandfatigue.com and www.fmaware.org. One of the most informative is Adrienne Dellwo's www.chronicfatigue.about.com. Besides her excellent up-to-date information and seemingly infinite knowledge of fibromyalgia, she has an outstanding blog and a lively discussion group. She also suffers from FMS, so you're getting firsthand knowledge here as well.

It is comforting to know you are not the only one with this pain, and just reading the blogs and past discussions will let you know that there is more help out there. There is the added benefit that others may have found helpful ideas for sleep or pain that may be helpful to you as well.

Options

There are many complementary and alternative options for fibromyalgia sufferers. That said, not all of them work for everyone. And there is no one treatment or combination of treatments that is perfect for every person with fibromyalgia. But each of the below listed therapy treatments has been shown to help the pain of fibromyalgia. So each person must decide which treatment or treatments he or she is most comfortable with. This, of course, means looking into each type of treatment in order to make an informed decision. Most use a combination of several of these therapies:

Acupressure

Acupuncture

Aromatherapy

Chiropractic Manipulation

Deep Breathing Exercises

Emotional Freedom Technique

Frequency Specific Microcurrent

Hydrotherapy

Hyperbaric Oxygen Therapy

Magnet Therapy

Massage Therapy

Meditation

Myofacial Pain Release

Nexalin Therapy

Physical Therapy

Reflexology

Reiki

Stretching

Swim/Water Therapy

Tai Chi

TENS Unit

Visualization

Walking

Yoga

When looking at this list—specifically acupressure, chiropractic manipulation, massage therapy, physical therapy, and reflexology—a question may arise.

"Are you crazy? I don't want anyone pushing on me. I hurt when *I* push on me. I hurt when *nothing* pushes on me!"

And the exercise therapies, such as tai chi, yoga, stretching, and even walking, may seem like they would add pain to an already painful body. But remember those endorphins. These pain-relieving chemicals that are released into your body, with all these touch and movement therapies, work like magic. These therapies also break up and release clumps of toxins that have attached to your muscles, and when they are released, much of your pain flows right out with them. Note how much the toe and ankle exercises help your pain in the morning.

And remember all the twelve million or more people with fibromyalgia who have come before you. They are using these therapies and finding blessed relief. That's where this list came from—from other people with fibromyalgia who have recommended them.

Where to Find These Therapies

All these therapies and more can be found and described in detail on the Internet, of course, but there are more personal and more hands-on means at your disposal. Large cities, medium-sized towns, and even small towns have libraries, YMCAs, health food stores, and hospital facilities.

Acupressure, acupuncture, massage therapy, and myofacial pain release therapy are much more available now than ever before and can usually be found in a telephone book or on a bulletin board or newsletter in a nearby health food store. Hyperbaric oxygen therapy, though not as well known, can usually be found by checking the bulletin board or newsletter at a health food store or by asking the manager or owner of that store. If they don't know of someone practicing the therapy, they can usually find out for you.

A good chiropractor is often found by word of mouth, but they are also listed in the phonebook.

Aromatherapy and magnet therapy can be learned from a practitioner found through your local health food store or through books at the local library or bookstore and, as stated, the Internet.

Deep breathing exercises, meditation, and visualization can be found in books, but consider finding a class through the YMCA, the local health food store, or even the library. There's a lot to be said for learning with a small group or class. The good energies are amplified, and this may lead to an excellent support group.

Physical therapy is usually found through your HCP or medical health care facility. Swim therapy can be accessed through there, as well as the local YMCA.

The YMCA may also have classes in yoga, tai chi, and stretching. As mentioned earlier, it is also possible to start out slowly by using a video at home.

Reflexology and Reiki healing therapies may be found through the local health food store bulletin board or newsletter, but some medical facilities have listings for these practitioners as well.

Walking, of course, can be done without any fee or special equipment other than good walking shoes, which is standard for anyone with fibromyalgia, along with loose, comfortable clothing. It can be done literally anywhere—outside or inside a mall in bad weather.

Electrical Therapies

There are two therapies, Frequency Specific Microcurrent[48] (FSM) and Nexalin Therapy,[49] that involve an electrical current in the millionth of an ampere (very, very low) and cannot even be felt by the patient. This tiny amount of current can be adjusted to match the exact amperage of the body's own electrical current to bring it back into alignment. Or it can be adjusted to neutralize a specific irregularity and bring it back into balance.

Each therapy requires a series of treatments for beneficial effect, which appears to be long-lasting. These therapies are not available in every hospital or clinic yet, but practitioners and clinics can be found on the Internet.

In FSM the practitioner uses a pad and/or vinyl gloves to apply the current to the patient's muscles. This increases the ATP energy in the muscles and eases pain.

In Nexalin therapy, while the patient relaxes in an easy chair (and usually naps), the practitioner applies three electrodes, which focus on normalizing the frequency of the hypothalamus.

The TENS unit, which is one thousand times greater in amperage than either of the above electrical therapies but still considered very low amp, is a portable unit, prescribed by a physician, where the patient can actually take the therapy along, wherever he or she goes, and use it as needed. It is a hand-held devise about the size of a small flashlight with an electrode on one end that is placed onto the painful area—hip, upper arm, back of the neck and shoulder area, lower back, etc. The transcutaneous electrical nerve stimulation (TENS) unit uses a low frequency of about eighty to ninety mega-hertz, which the user can adjust in several ways, including strength of the electrical current, how long each pulse width is, and/or whether it is continuous or pulsating. Because this device is a prescription item, you will need to consult your HCP for more info. You can also check them out online   Google "TENS unit."

Alternate Therapy

Emotional Freedom Technique (EFT), commonly called "tapping," uses only your own fingers. No external objects needed. It is a form of needle-less acupuncture where you tap on specific meridian points with your own fingertips with the intention of releasing blocked emotional, painful energies, clearing the pathway for free-flowing energies. This therapy has helped millions for a huge number of concerns, ranging from emotional trauma, depression, back pain, migraines, PTSD, and much more. Doctors, psychologists, physical therapists, chiropractors, and all manner of the healing profession have used this therapy in their practices. But you can do it too. It takes only minutes to learn, and instructions can be downloaded for free online at www.EFTUniverse.com, or you can Google "Emotional Freedom Technique" and go to any of the many Web sites available. Information can also be found in your favorite bookstores.

Supplemental Options

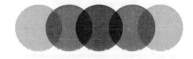

Natural supplements, vitamins, and herbs have been, and are still being, used successfully all over the world. For example, peppermint oil (not the flavoring) is still used to calm nausea, flatulence (gas), and heartburn. Basil is not only a very tasty herb, but it is also known for easing stress, helping the immune system, and aiding digestion. Vitamin C is well known for helping the immune system and minimizing colds.

Because the human body naturally attempts to heal itself, a chronically ill body will use every vitamin, mineral, enzyme, antioxidant, etc., in this attempt, and it will use them at an alarming rate. And so these must be replenished every day in the form of healthy, whole, natural (unprocessed) foods that have retained all their vitamins, minerals, enzymes, antioxidants, etc. When this is not possible or practical due to seasonal factors or poor farmland issues, natural supplements, vitamins, and herbs can help.

Herbs and Supplements

These may well be among the most helpful treatments for fibromyalgia pain and restful sleep. Some of the most beneficial herbs and supplements for fibromyalgia recommended by medical doctors, naturopaths, alternative healers, researchers, and fibromyalgia sufferers themselves are: Omega 3, magnesium, malic acid, alpha lipoic acid, vitamin D, CoQ10, eleuthero, rhodiola, Sam-e, and immune supporters like garlic extract, olive leaf extract, oil of oregano, and sleep helpers like 5-HTP or melatonin. Then, of course, there are the basics of a good high quality multivitamin and water.

Note: Before taking any supplements, check
with your health care provider (HCP). Always
tell your HCP of any medications or supplements you are currently taking.

Buying Supplements

When purchasing any supplements, it's wise to avoid
the dollar store variety and those of that ilk. On the
other hand, just because a supplement is at a high-
end price, don't automatically assume it is top quality. Consider checking with www.ConsumerLab.com
first. It's true that there are many reliable, well-known
supplement brands out there, but this third party,
independent testing lab has made it their business to
keep the public informed of safe and reliable supplements. This testing group regularly conducts random
tests on hundreds of supplements and herbs then
publishes their findings online for all the public to see.

This is a subscription site, which also has a great
free newsletter. The small fee for joining allows not
only access to each and every detailed finding on all
the chosen supplements but also allows access to a
wonderful science-based library and medical encyclopedia to find out more about the supplements you are

looking for. They are also the first ones to send you information about any recalls. All in all, this is one of those informative sites that are considered priceless.

A number of popular brands consistently show positive ratings, such as Carlson's, Country Life, GNC, Nature Made, Nature's Bounty, Puritan's Pride, Spring Valley, Swanson's, The Vitamin Shoppe, Twin Lab, etc. However, each product is tested individually every year, so it is always good to check with the site for specifics.

List of Fibromyalgia Supplements

Omega 3

These essential fatty acids are indeed *essential* for our overall health. But our body doesn't make them, so we must add them to our diet. As it turns out, Americans are way out of balance in the proper essential fatty acids. Clearly, as shown the previous chapter we have more than enough Omega 6 (inflammatory) fatty acids in our current Western diet. Even *more* clearly, we need to *add* Omega 3 to bring back the proper balance, in order to end the inflammation, ease pain, lower blood pressure, balance mood, bolster the immune system, and much more. Please refer to "Edible Aggravators" for more valuable information and recommended dosage.

Magnesium

Magnesium helps ease muscle pain, contributes immeasurably to energy production, and activates enzymes to aid in absorption of calcium, vitamin D, potassium, copper, and more. In fact magnesium is involved in more than 325 biological functions, including the relaxation of muscles and cells. Yet most Americans can be classified as having magnesium insufficiency![50] Calcium contracts; magnesium relaxes. If your muscles contract more than they relax, you are in pain!

For fibromyalgia and chronic fatigue syndrome, Dr. Teitelbaum recommends 250 mg two or three times a day of absorbable magnesium, such as magnesium glycinate,[51] magnesium citrate, magnesium aspartate, or magnesium malate. The popular magnesium oxide, widely found in drugstores, is inexpensive and helpful if you need a good laxative, but its absorption rate leaves a lot to be desired. The idea here is *not* for magnesium to pass through but to be absorbed into your bloodstream and muscle tissue, where it's needed.

Topical magnesium, such as Epsom salts, magnesium chloride bath salts, or sea salt, is also effective. These products are inexpensive and can be found in any health food store, local drugstore, or grocery store. One cupful or more of these salts dissolved into a very warm bath will absorb into your skin and then into your bloodstream, delivering blessed relief to your cells and muscles in a warm, soothing twenty minutes. It's almost as good as going to an expensive mineral bath or health spa!

Malic Acid

Malate is a naturally occurring compound in the body that plays an important role in the production of energy. However, as we age or become ill, our natural production of this compound is greatly reduced.

The supplement of malic acid is an acid derived from fruit, mostly apples, that helps the body to make energy in the cells, even under low oxygen conditions. Over and above its ability to raise energy levels and ease pain,[52] malic acid also helps remove excessively high levels of aluminum and other undesirable metals in the body and most especially in the brain. A dosage of 1200 mg to 2400 mg per day has been used in clinical tests. [53]

Alpha Lipoic Acid

This supplement has been used for over thirty years in Europe to relieve diabetic nerve pain. It is also excellent for fibromyalgic nerve pain, including numb and tingling hands and fingers and burning, prickling skin so sensitive to touch.

It is also an excellent super-antioxidant. Because it is both water and fat soluble, it can work throughout the body. It also cleans up vitamin C (water soluble) and vitamin E (fat soluble) and puts them back to work as antioxidants on their own.

According to the University of Maryland Medical Center, the recommended dose for diabetic neuropathy (nerve pain) is 800 mg per day in divided doses.[54] Half that dosage, 400 mg in divided doses, works well for nerve pain caused by other factors, including fibromyalgia. After several months, a maintenance dose of 200–300 mg works quite well.

Antioxidants of any kind are extremely important for health. All illnesses can benefit from antioxidant use because they fight free radicals, which add insult to injury when it comes to illness, whether chronic, degenerative, or simply the common cold.[55]

The Importance of Antioxidants

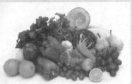 Antioxidants are crucial in helping a chronically ill body. Not only do they help boost and rebuild the immune system, but they actually *prevent* and *reverse* damage caused by free radicals.

Free radicals are *not* fibro-friendly. In fact, they are linked to many chronic and degenerative diseases, including fibromyalgia, chronic fatigue syndrome, rheumatoid arthritis, heart disease, even cancer. When free radicals are allowed to build up to a dangerous tipping point in the body, they begin running amok, damaging the DNA within the cells, even destroying and killing cells!

Antioxidants come to the rescue. Visualize a flying red cape here! Fortunately, they are abundant and easy to obtain, unlike other superheroes. Antioxidants are found in fresh whole foods, like fruits and veggies, nuts, legumes, and whole grains. They're available in supplements, like alpha lipoic acid, CoQ10, bilberry, garlic extract, grape seed extract, green tea, quercetin, zinc, and others. Most herbs, such as sage, rosemary, basil, and thyme, along with garlic and onion, contain antioxidants. Vitamins A, C, E, and selenium (ACEs), which are always found in a multivitamin, are antioxidants.

Antioxidants are abundant in the new fruit juices like açai, mangostene, noni, and pomegranate. They are found in dark chocolate, with even more available in the unprocessed dark chocolate delicacy, Xoçai chocolate.

And, of course, the fresh fruits and veggies in a capsule, Juice Plus+ is loaded with antioxidants. These capsules have the added benefit of including natural enzymes and probiotics too.

It's important to know that most antioxidants are specialists, each working in a different area of the body. So it's better to take a moderate amount of several kinds of antioxidants rather than a lot of any specific one.

> Taking antioxidants throughout the day, every day, is an excellent way to help your body now and to help your future health as well.

Vitamin D

Vitamin D helps ease pain. It is also necessary to enable calcium's absorption. Everyone who lives in the northern two-thirds of the United States needs extra vitamin D, especially in the winter. Seniors and those with darker pigmented skin need extra vitamin D because their body makes an insufficient amount on its own from the sun. According to WebMD, recent studies have shown that insufficient vitamin D is linked to osteoporosis, breast cancer, heart disease, depression, autoimmune diseases, high blood pressure, and more. Ask your HCP to check your vitamin D levels. You may be quite surprised by the results. Newer recommended doses, especially in the winter and in northern latitudes, are 1,000 IU—5,000 IU per day.[56]

CoQ10

Co-enzyme Q10 is found in the mitochondria of each cell. It is a natural energy producer involved in a wide range of the body's systems, particularly in heart function. It's also a powerful antioxidant. This natural co-enzyme is abundant in infancy but decreases steadily as we age. Because it is involved in energy production and the well-being of our DNA, it is good to replenish this important co-enzyme as we become older, especially if we become chronically ill.

Because CoQ10 is not water soluble, it must be taken with an oil in order to be properly absorbed. Some brands of this enzyme include a small amount of vitamin E to aid in its absorption. The University of Maryland Medical Center recommends adult doses of 30 200 mg per day. [57]

Eleuthero

Formerly known as Siberian ginseng, this herb has been used for centuries in Russia, China, and other Eastern countries. Traditionally it had been used for colds and flu and to increase energy, vitality, and stamina. This is an adaptogenic herb that helps the body adapt to various kinds of physical and emotional stress, such as heat, cold, exertion, sleep deprivation, and hormonal fluctuations. It is helpful in promoting energy and aids in supporting the immune system. The recommended dose, according to the University of Maryland Medical Center, is a standardized extract of 100–200 mg two times daily.[58]

Rhodiola

Rhodiola is similar in action to eleuthero, even though it's a wholly different plant. Also an adaptogen, it has been used in Scandinavia and Russia for centuries, where it has been the subject of major written research since the late 1700s. It has been used for all of the same conditions as eleuthero, including depression and mental fatigue. Dosage is commonly 200–600 mg per day. [59]

Some people will alternate one month of eleuthero, the next with rhodiola, in order to prevent the body from adapting too comfortably to one or the other. This keeps the action of each herb fresh.

Sam-e

Sam-e, short for S-adenosylmethionine, is present in every living cell in the body and is involved in many biochemical processes. Sam-e is not found in food; it is produced by the body, but as we age our levels of production decline.

The supplement Sam-e has been shown to improve the pain, fatigue, mood, and morning stiffness of fibromyalgia. Sam-e is also used to treat depression, chronic fatigue syndrome, osteoarthritis, ADHD, and more.

In Europe, where Sam-e is classified as an antidepressant and is a prescription medication, it has been used successfully for many years to treat depression, arthritis, chronic fatigue syndrome, and fibromyalgia. In the United States it is sold over the counter.

Sam-e is not meant to be used with other antidepressant medications, nor should it to be used by people with bipolar disorder. Please consult your HCP for suggested use.

Recommended dosage of Sam-e, as suggested by the University of Maryland Medical Center, is 400 mg twice a day for six weeks for fibromyalgia; then take a two-week break and consult your HCP for further directions. Different doses are recommended for arthritis, depression, etc.[60]

Garlic Extract, Olive Leaf Extract, Oil of Oregano

These herbs provide potent immune system support and powerful antioxidant support. They help fight off bacteria, viruses, and fungus, which is a must for FMS sufferers because a simple infection or a cold can amplify *all* of their fibromyalgia symptoms.

Garlic extract[61] and olive leaf extract[62] may have the added benefit of helping to maintain a healthy heart and circulatory system. Both raise the HDL (good cholesterol) levels and decrease LDL (bad cholesterol) levels, and both are known to lower blood pressure and act as blood thinners. Neither should be used prior to surgery or if Warfarin has been prescribed.

Oil of oregano[63] is derived from the wild oregano species, different from the oregano in the grocery store. It is a powerful antimicrobial, antiviral, antifungal, antiparasitic, anti-inflammatory, and painkiller.

All are available at your local health food stores and most drugstores. For each of these immune boosters, follow the directions on the label for appropriate dosage.

5-HTP or Melatonin

The amino acid 5-hydroxytryptophan (5-HTP) is another compound that is produced in the body, but as we age or become ill, this production slows way down. 5-HTP helps the body produce serotonin, which has a positive effect on mood, sleep, anxiety, and pain sensation. It has been shown to improve sleep quality and reduce pain, stiffness, anxiety, and depression in fibromyalgia sufferers.[64] The University of Maryland Medical Center recommends 50 mg one to three times a day.

Melatonin is a hormone secreted by the pineal gland that regulates the biological rhythms associated with light and dark—the circadian rhythm. In other words, it governs the sleep cycle. Melatonin levels also become lower as we age, which is why sleep cycles often become disrupted or change as we get older.[65] Melatonin is especially helpful for people with jetlag or night workers who have a mixed up day/night schedule.

Dr. Teitelbaum says that to restore the normal amount of melatonin for most people requires only 300 mcg (0.3 mg), which is the amount normally produced by the body. When using much more than that, such as found on the shelf in most stores (usually 3 mg, which is *ten times* his recommended amount), there is a tendency to work in the reverse for some people and keep them wired because of its effects on other hormones.[66]

Ask your HCP if either of these supplements would be right for you. *Neither* 5-HTP nor melatonin should be taken with an antidepressant, a selective serotonin reuptake inhibitor (SSRI), selective serotonin, and norepinephrine reuptake inhibitor (SNRI) or a monoamine oxidase inhibitor (MAOI).

Multivitamin

A good, high quality multivitamin can help tremendously. This will ensure that your body gets the all-important, pain-relieving B vitamins and folic acid your body requires, along with the selenium, niacin, biotin, zinc, and all the other essential vitamins and minerals that are so crucial for a body in pain. Check with www.ConsumerLab.com for a good quality multivitamin. The modern Western diet is sorely lacking in the most basic of essential nutrients due to overuse of soil and so much processing and quick meals, frozen and otherwise. Give yourself the edge needed to rebuild your most basic resources.

Another plus for multivitamins is that according to the June 1, 2009, issue of the *Journal of Clinical Nutrition*, multivitamin use in women was found to increase the telomeres (end regions of the DNA) by a full 5.1 percent, compared to those who didn't use multivitamins.[67] So what does that mean? Longer telomeres indicate healthy DNA—definitely a good thing because short telomeres are associated with fraying ends and damage to the DNA, chromosome damage, and aging.

Note: The researchers suspect this benefit may stem from the antioxidant properties found in the multi from the B vitamins, zinc, and numerous other ingredients within the multi that work as antioxidants, wiping out free radicals.

Water

Think of water as a lubricant for your dry, stiff, aching muscles, tendons, ligaments, joints, and organs. Rehydrating these and all your body parts is invaluable to helping pain. In fact, Don Colbert, M.D., author of *The Seven Pillars of Health*, calls water the most important foundational aspect of health.[68]

Water helps eliminate acid wastes that build up in a chronically ill body. And if you are retaining fluids, it is important to flush out the old, stale, possibly toxic fluids that are being held in your tissues.

Water is especially important if you are taking supplements, herbs, or medications. Water enables the supplements to flow freely through your bloodstream and be moved along throughout your muscles and other tissues, delivering their payload.

Only water counts. Coffee and soft drinks are diuretics, actually causing you to lose water.

How much water should you drink? For healthy people, at least eight full eight-ounce glasses of water per day is usually recommended. But for those who are chronically ill, even more is needed. Jane Oelke, N.D., Ph.D., recommends drinking "one-half your weight in ounces of water."[69] So, for example, if you weigh one hundred and fifty pounds, you would need seventy-five ounces of water per day. She also recommends spreading out that amount of water throughout the day—it's easier on the kidneys.

The point is that water serves a purpose in the body—it is, in fact, absolutely essential for the body to function properly. Coffee, soft drinks, and alcohol actually impair many of those functions, especially when used in excess.

What To Do For You

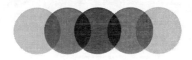

Helping yourself is the very best thing you can do. In fact, you are the *only* one who can effectively treat your fibromyalgia.

The very first thing to do is find the right doctor *for you*—a doctor you can trust and who will work *with* you. One who will *gladly* answer questions and be willing to explain why this or that treatment is for you. If your family doctor is not familiar with fibromyalgia or has no experience in its treatment, he may refer you to a rheumatologist. Or you may choose to seek out a HCP in the integrative medical field, an osteopath, or naturopath. Many with fibromyalgia have a separate doctor for their fibromyalgia symptoms—a specialist as it were—one who is familiar with the myriad of different presentations of this particular condition and knows what to look for.

Let your fingers do the walking and call someone from a local support group. Ask for names of their favorite doctors. Your local health food store may have information about knowledgeable HCPs in this area. You can also go to http://www.wellness.com/find/integrative%20doctor and click on your state, then your town, or go to http://www.locateadoc.com/doctors/integrative-medicine.html, or Google "Integrative Medical Physician."

Help Yourself

Learn everything you can about fibromyalgia online, in books, in videos, or from support groups. Arm yourself with information. The following chapter, "Bountiful Resources," is filled with choices. Acquire enough knowledge about the subject to know what questions to ask your doctor, to know what to look for, and to know what to avoid.

Journaling

Keep a journal or make notes in your iPod, Blackberry, or laptop. Write down the date and time a flare-up occurs. Then write down possible aggravators that could have brought on the flare. Think back to what you had been doing or eating earlier or the day before. Connect the dots.

You might want to do an elimination test on nightshades, aspartame, MSG, sugar, coffee, or soft drinks. Note the day you begin and what symptoms you're experiencing at the time. Then, each day, note any changes in symptoms you may experience while not using the substance. Note everything. Keep track. This is for *you* and *your* healing.

Write down any medications you are taking, when you began, the dosage and any effects, for good or ill. This information is invaluable to your doctor. If you write it all down, you won't forget it when you have your next appointment in two or three weeks. This will let your HCP know if the dosage needs to be raised or lowered or if a different medication is needed. Arm yourself with the facts. In print.

Stress Relief

Learn some stress relief techniques. Prevent stress before it begins by recognizing your limitations. It has been shown that most people with fibromyalgia are overachievers and/or people pleasers. These are good things to be sure, but not at the expense of your health.

Stress amplifies fibromyalgic symptoms. *Create* time to be good to yourself—every single day. Relaxation, prayer, meditation, doing something that brings you joy—all these are essential. All of these can neutralize stress.

Emotional Freedom Technique can also help in relieving stress. Deep breathing can relieve stress. Certain supplements can relieve stress. Do whatever works for you. You *must* de-stress.

Pacing

Pace yourself realistically for your condition. You may have to learn to say "no" gracefully. You cannot be all things to all people all the time. Fibromyalgia is a part of your life now, and you must pace yourself. You already know that when you push yourself to get everything done in one day, pain will set you back drastically for the next *three* days. Activity, rest, activity, rest, even on the good days—*especially* on the good days—is crucial.

Temporary Relief

Sometimes temporary relief can come from your local drugstore, Target, or Wal-Mart in the form of ointments, creams, hot or cold packs, magnetic wrist or knee wraps, or bath salts.

Epsom salts, portable foot or neck massagers, and Salonpas Pain Patches are helpful. Capsaicin ointment, or roll-on liquid, applied topically, is said to neutralize that pain-making substance P. All of these are readily available to temporarily help pain.

Diphenhydramine HCL at 25 mg, e.g. Benedryl, or other sleep aids your HCP may approve of: eye drops for dry eye and acidophilus for stomach issues. These are only a few examples of pain and symptom relievers that are easily attainable everywhere. But you must make the effort. Ask your HCP if any of these may be of help in your case.

Experiment

Learn what works for you. Try new therapies. Maybe reflexology, massage therapy, or acupuncture will appeal to you. Walking, tai chi, or stretching may be your cup of tea. Take a bath in Epsom salts with an aromatherapy beeswax candle and soothing music. Often your own body in the form of a gut feeling will tell you what you need to do. Drink more water. Read up on the list of supplements and choose which ones you believe may help you. Then talk to your HCP. Your body is not the enemy here. It's simply telling you change is needed. Listen to it.

Dr. D.A. Williams and Dr. M. Carey of the University of Michigan Health System share the most valuable tip of all[70]:

> Pain is associated with negative emotions such as sadness, frustration, and irritability. When people are in pain and also have these emotions, the pain becomes worse. That is because these emotions are processed in the same area of the brain, as is pain.
>
> Research has shown that pain decreases when people experience more positive emotions.

So Do Something that Brings You Joy!

Go fly a kite. Go fishing. Skip a stone on a pond. Take a walk in the park, and watch a squirrel run up a tree. Go out and buy the most huggable stuffed animal you can find. Read a good heart-warming book. Watch an uplifting movie. Work with your hands—do a craft or work a jigsaw puzzle. Play with your pet. Wear colorful clothes. Bring some light and color into your workplace and your home—bring in some upbeat music while you're at it. Go to the park and feed the ducks. Learn to dance. Learn tai chi. Smile. Treat yourself to a manicure, a pedicure, a new hairstyle, or a massage. Take an aromatherapy bath in the middle of the afternoon, complete with surrounding candles. Cultivate your sense of humor—read a joke book. Build a mini-snowman and set him on your front step. Redecorate a room—throw a splash of color here and there. Work a Sudoku puzzle or a crossword puzzle. Volunteer at a hospital. Volunteer to read books to children at your local library. Blow bubbles—pink bubble gum, remember? Buy a bottle of bubbles and blow bubbles for your dog! Smile. Buy a yo-yo. Go to the beach or the river and collect pretty stones. Go out and play in your garden. Start a window garden. Pick up a paintbrush or some crayons and draw. Start a journal. Write down all the fun things *you* can think of.

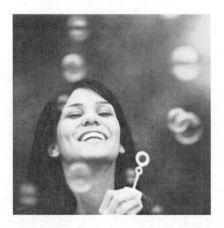

Lift your life and heal the pain.

List of Things to Do

Fibromyalgia is not a one-treatment-fits-all kind of syndrome. Arm yourself with information. Then get moving ... literally. Bit by bit, build up your strength, five minutes at a time. See your osteopath, naturopath, or integrative medical physician; go to your local health food store; go to the library; check out your local YMCA and buy a swimsuit. Join a support group. Sign up for a newsletter to get the latest information on any one of the fibromyalgia Web sites. Find your balance of exercise, rest, play, and work. You must be the biggest part of your treatment.

Depending on which Web site you consult, there are seven million, ten million, or twelve million Americans who have fibromyalgia. With the numbers growing at this rate of speed, more and more researchers are hard at work looking for a cure.

But maybe a *cure* isn't necessarily what's needed. Maybe it's change that's needed. Change of our lifestyle, our eating habits, our outlook, or our ability to be at peace with our body and those bodies around us.

Find something that makes your heart
shout for joy—and then do it!

Bountiful Resources

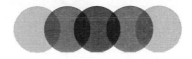

There are a multitude of resources available for finding out more about fibromyalgia and how to manage it, as well as finding out about the newest and latest research. Some of them are: your local library; health food store; health care facility; Web sites; magazines such as *Arthritis Today* and others; your local YMCA; and even the phonebook under "Physical Therapists," "Pain Management," or "Physicians-Arthritis" to name a few. The below listed sites, books, and videos are a few places to start:

Fibromyalgia Web Sites

1. http://chronicfatigue.about.com. This is Adrienne
    Dellwo's great fibromyalgia/CFS Web site. She
    has fibromyalgia and chronic fatigue syndrome
    and goes to all lengths to be certain she has the
    latest information on everything from new medi-
    cations, to new treatments, to handy "thinga-
    majigs" to make life a bit easier for everyone who's
    in her boat. Click on everything—she is a gold
    mine of information! She has an excellent blog,
    a lively online discussion group, and an excellent
    free newsletter.

2. www.endfatigue.com. This is Dr. Jacob
    Teitelbaum's Web site. Click on everything. Dr.
    Teitelbaum has literally hundreds of articles on
    fibromyalgia and chronic fatigue syndrome and
    videos so you can watch him explain what's up.
    There are lists and descriptions of his treatment
    protocol for the SHIN program. He also has
    listings of supplements and even a store to buy
    them. You'll find a discussion board and a free
    newsletter here as well.

3. www.fmaware.com. This is the Web site for the National Fibromyalgia Association. This is one great resource center. Hundreds of articles, a store, an online community, research information, a fibromyalgia professional resource center, and a "find a support group" link.

4. www.prohealth.com. This site has a bounty of information including the latest research from medical schools and facilities and papers by a large number of physicians whose practice is focused on helping those with fibromyalgia and chronic fatigue syndrome. There is a great store where their supplements have been third party independently tested. There is a message board and chat room and "find a support group" links and more.

Condition Specific Web Sites

1. www.womentowomen.com. This site is geared to women's issues. Dr. Marcelle Pick, OB/GYN NP, is a naturopathic physician who has gathered together several physicians who specialize in complicated or difficult women's issues, such

as fibromyalgia, menopause, hypothyroidism, and celiac disease all combined in one person, for example. Though their clinic has been located in Yarmouth, Maine, for the past twenty-five years, they have branched out to the Internet. They have an 800 number where you can ask questions for your particular case and even set up your own personal program of healing. Type "fibromyalgia" in their search box, and you will come up with acres of great information.

2. www.glutenfreeworks.com. This Web site is devoted to those who are learning or those who are old hands at gluten-free living. It is a great resource for both. Definitions, thorough explanations of non-celiac gluten sensitivity and celiac disease, as well as a symptom guide, information about testing and treatment can be found here, along with recipes, foods to watch out for, or changes in listed "safe" foods and much more. A list of gluten-free foods and gluten substitutes helps greatly. Sign up for regular updates!

3. www.foodintol.com. Deborah Manners is the host of this excellent Web site. Here you will find information about all sorts of sensitivities, including gluten sensitivity, lactose intolerance, yeast sensitivity, fructose sensitivity, and wheat intolerance, which is different than gluten sensitivity. Click on "Content Index," and a whole world opens up. If you ever had questions about or suspected you might have a food intolerance, this is the place to come. Everything is explained thoroughly and clearly. Then she provides help—through diet, elimination, substitution, and more. Become a member for free, and there are even more doors of information opened for you.

Medical Facilities and Their Web Site

1. University of Maryland Medical Center, Baltimore, Maryland. **www.umm.edu**. Type "Fibromyalgia"; click on "go." This will take you to a listing of thirty-five to forty of the latest articles on fibromyalgia, where you can choose which one you'd like to read. **www.umm.edu/altmed**.

This will take you to the "Complementary and Alternative Index, Medical Reference Site." If you click on "condition," you can choose the illness you want to learn about: fibromyalgia, chronic fatigue, hypothyroidism, Lyme disease, Raynaud's syndrome, or any other condition that you may be sharing with fibromyalgia. You can click on "herb" then scroll down to the herb you'd like to read about. Or "Supplement" or "Treatment" or "Side-effects" or "Interactions." This site is a literal bounty of complementary medical information.

2. University of Michigan Health System/Chronic Pain and Fatigue Research Center, Ann Arbor, Michigan. **www.med.umich.edu/painresearch/patients/index.htm**. When you arrive at this pain and fatigue research site, you will read about the latest studies and research being done on pain. There are hyperlinks to "Advice to Patients," "Learn about Self-Management Skills," "Participate in Pain Research Study," and "Learn About Fibromyalgia." This is the

research center where Dr. Clauw and his team proved via fMRI that fibromyalgia pain is real.

3. National Institute of Arthritis and Musculoskeletal and Skin Diseases (NIAMS), Division of National Institute of Health (NIH), Bethesda, Maryland. **www.niams.nih.gov.** Click on "F" then "fibromyalgia." Here you will find a thorough description of fibromyalgia and answers to many questions. And for the scientifically minded, you can click on "Clinical Trials" and search for any specific testing being done now, or you can browse until you find something applicable to your case. You can click on "Journal Articles," and you will be swept away to Pubmed.org, where you will be able to read all the actual medical abstracts then the full in-depth article written by the doctors, Ph.D.s, scientists, nutritionists, microbiologists, etc.

4. National Center For Complementary and Alternative Medicine (NCCAM), Division of NIH, Bethesda, Maryland. **http://nccam.nih. gov.** This Web site has a full description of nearly

all of the complementary and alternative medical (CAM) therapies for all kinds of illnesses. You'll find full descriptions and uses for acupuncture, chiropractic, massage, Reiki, reflexology, yoga, tai chi, herbs, supplements, magnet therapy, and more. *And* you'll find it in Spanish too. Type "Fibromyalgia" in the search box, and you'll not only find information on fibromyalgia but also on the numerous CAM therapies that have been shown to help fibromyalgia.

Healthy Web Sites

1. www.WebMD.com. Click on "fibromyalgia." Or you can click on any other condition or supplement or diet or women's health or men's health issues. It is an enormously popular medical information Web site for good reason. Used by patients and doctors alike.

2. www.healthy.net. This is a natural and integrative medical Web site. Contributors to this site include Dr. Jacob Teitelbaum; Nan Fuchs, Ph.D.; Dr. Elson Haas; and many more. Alternative

medicine, integrative medicine, homeopathic medicine, natural medicine, nutritional, and herbal therapies are addressed here. Your spiritual and emotional health are addressed here, as well as your physical health. There is a free newsletter, a bookstore, a discussion board, recipes, links to "Find a Practitioner" and "Discount Lab Tests," and much more. Another gold mine of information and help for healing.

3. www.Drugs.com. This is an excellent informational site not only for prescription drugs, their side effects, interactions, and precautions but also for natural products, like herbs and supplements.

4. www.PatiChandlerJuicePlus.com. This is Pati Chandler's home site of Juice Plus+, where you can find a list of products for adults and children, information about antioxidants, how the product is made, the medical abstracts, the science behind the benefits of the products, and the latest updated research.

5. http//xocai.com. This is the home page of Xoçai Healthy Chocolate, where you can find

a list of their products, the science behind the healthy chocolate, contact information for dealers in the USA, Hong Kong, Sweden, Australia, the Netherlands, and more.

Electrical Frequency Therapies

1. www.frequencyspecific.com. Click on the video to find out more.

2. www.NexalinTherapy.com. Click on the video to find out more.

3. www.tensunits.com. Click on the video to find out more.

Wikipedia

This is an excellent source for hyperlinks to more information.

http://en.wikipedia.org/wiki/Fibromyalgia. Click on everything blue, including the reference numbers—134 at last count. These will take you to the medical references and abstracts, medical journal entries, and scientific studies for even *more* information.

Books

- *Fibromyalgia and Chronic Myofacial Pain Syndrome: A Survival Manual*, 1996. By Devin Starlanyl and Mary Ellen Copeland, M.S., M.A.

- *From Fatigued To Fantastic*, 2007. By Jacob Teitelbaum, M.D.

- *Natural Choices For Fibromyalgia*, 2001. By Jane Oelke, N.D., Ph.D.

- *The Everything Health Guide to Fibromyalgia*, 2006. By Winnie Yu and Michael M. McNett, M.D.

- *The Seven Pillars of Health—The Natural Way to Better Health For Life*, 2007. By Don Colbert, M.D.

- *Alternative Medicine—The Definitive Guide*, 2002. By Burton Goldberg.

Videos

This is a list of videos for purposeful movement. Movement, remember, is not for strength training or weight loss here; rather, it is a necessity to increase circulation of blood, oxygen, and nutrients like magnesium, etc., to get to your muscles and for creating those pain-relieving endorphins!

- *Gentle Tai Chi* from Terra Entertainment (in a seated position)
- *Moving to Mozart* with Ann Smith
- *Qigong for Beginners* with Daisy Lee and Francesco Garripoli
- *Stretching for Seniors* with Ann Smith
- *Tai Chi for Beginners* with Paul Lam
- *Tai Chi for Arthritis* with Paul Lam
- *Tai Chi for Back Pain* with Paul Lam

Online Video

www.FibroKnowledge.com. This is an informational video online, produced by Pfizer Incorporated for physicians and patients. For those who have loved ones who would rather watch a video than read a book on the subject, this is an excellent interactive video covering what fibromyalgia is, what symptoms are common, how it's diagnosed, and how it's treated.

If your HCP, friends, or family members are not familiar with fibromyalgia, this will cover the basics.

Fibromyalgia Video

Wellness Solutions for Fibromyalgia. This video is put together by the Mayo Clinic and GAIAM, a company focused on natural health and healing. You'll find copious amounts of valuable information on fibromyalgia, integrative medicine, diet, meditation, yoga, and other methods of helping with pain and exhaustion.

The Author's Fibromyalgia Story

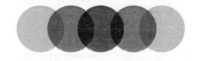

My journcy with fibromyalgia began in the winter of 1998. It started out with a cold that, over the course of two months, turned into a bad case of bronchitis, which turned into a severe cough that bruised and ultimately crackcd a rib—a hairline fracture, the chiropractor said. With all this severe coughing wracking my body for weeks, not only did my ribs take the hit, but also my neck and shoulders, my head, my chest, my back, my arms—in fact, my entire body felt like it had been tumbling around in a cement mixer ... *with* all the aggregate chunks of concrete and stones beating on me!

I was exhausted, totally wrung out. After three months, the bronchitis was gone and the cough was finally a bad memory, although I was still wearing a rib brace, but I still experienced all the body pain, exhaustion, and weakness I had felt from the first week of the episode. I went to our local Medpoint, where the doctor told me it was just taking longer than usual to snap back. After all, it had been quite a severe case of bronchitis.

During these months I had taken one whole week off work. Fortunately, my job with the Department of Natural Resources (DNR) required lots of time in the car alone, lots of time with salmon and trout (and small mouth bass and walleye), and a minimal amount of time with people. So, although my bronchitis had raged on, even after that week off, I was not going around infecting others. Evidently fish don't get bronchitis. But I came home each day utterly exhausted, unable to do anything but rest. And even *that* hurt.

The cough that had lingered on and on finally left, but months later why did my body still feel like I was in that cement mixer? Why was my body still so weak I could hardly hold a cup of coffee or lift my leg to get in the car? Why did I nearly fall on the floor in pain when I woke up every morning? The questions kept coming and coming with each additional symptom. And they *did* add up, one *more* thing after another after another.

Things were getting worse, not better. I thought my mind was going the way of the dodo. I couldn't remember things. I lost things. I couldn't remember what I was going to say or even *how to say it*. I would lose words! I seemed so clumsy. I dropped things and bumped into things all the time. The kitchen doorway seemed to be a favorite miscalculation. I had a constant bruise on my left shoulder from running into the doorjamb all the time. I stubbed my toe on the bed frame regularly or the computer chair wheels. I stumbled over nothing—cracks in the hardwood floor or a throw rug that I have been living with for years! I was getting scared.

And then there was this peculiar "Princess and the Pea" syndrome where a wrinkle in my nightgown or my sheet was so uncomfortable that I couldn't get settled to sleep. A fold in my sock felt like I was walking on a rock. My body was so sensitive I could feel *everything* that wasn't right. A bunched-up shirt under a sweatshirt was a nightmare to straighten out. Sitting in the car with my slacks bunched up was impossible to bear. It felt like I was sitting on a mound of stones. It hurt!

I couldn't sit longer than fifteen minutes anyway because my body would begin to hurt all over, so I'd stand up. Then my hips, legs, and feet would begin to hurt after ten minutes, so I'd sit down. After fifteen minutes, I got up again. Then I'd sit down again. All day long! Lying down only helped for about twenty minutes because I had to move to a different position there too. If I did fall asleep, I hurt like crazy when I woke up.

Lights bothered me. I spent nearly all my time wearing sunglasses—even in the house. The TV seemed ultra-bright—my computer screen, the light over the kitchen sink, never mind the sunlight outside—my eyes burned and watered, and my face hurt from squinting. Loud noises seemed piercing and reverberated in my head—my ears would ring and hurt for the next fifteen minutes after a single loud noise. Needless to say, I didn't make it to many of my grandchildren's basketball, football, or cheerleading events during that time.

I would eat a half a sandwich and become so bloated I felt as if I was going to explode! I tried a

Carnation Instant Breakfast, just for the vitamins, and became so bloated and uncomfortable I felt you could roll me to the bathroom! I was miserable for the next hour or two. And to top it all off, I was spending an inordinate amount of time in the bathroom. Every time I turned around I had to go—morning, noon, and nighttime too.

Things got progressively worse, and after six months of this I finally had to leave the best job of my life with the DNR. Depression set in firmly. And I was *still* getting worse, not better.

I had come to the point where I thought I was going crazy. I thought I would never be able to work again or even write again. I couldn't sit long enough, and I couldn't focus. I couldn't even *think* normally. Truthfully, I didn't care enough about anything except how much I hurt. I was certain I was going to be in a wheelchair with MS soon and I wouldn't be able to get into my own home. Was it carpal tunnel and nerve damage and Alzheimer's and Crohn's disease too? All *kind*s of things ran through my head. Depressed? You bet. My life had changed absolutely. I was scared to tell anyone *all* my symptoms; *no one* had this many symptoms. They'd think I was nuts.

Someone finally recommended Dr. Bhatt, an osteopath. I had never been to one of those, but I figured I had nothing to lose. I was ready to try anyone. I had decided to tell him only a few of my symptoms. I didn't have a regular family doctor back then, so I figured if he thought I was crazy, I would never have to see him again.

The visions of being in a wheelchair with MS or in surgery for carpal tunnel syndrome or in a nursing home for fifty-two-year-olds with Alzheimer's were constantly on my mind. I had gone to Dr. Bhatt out of desperation; I wanted him to get rid of my pain *and* all the other malfunctions.

After describing the pain I had been experiencing for the prior six months, he finally asked me how I felt when I woke in the morning. When I told him, he gently laid his finger on my skin near my clavicle. The pain he evoked brought me to tears as I pulled away from him.

He raised his eyebrows, nodded his head, and said, "Uh-huh."

Through my tears and pain, I said, "What uh-huh?"

He somehow convinced me to sit there (reluctantly) while he proceeded to lay his finger on seventeen more tender points. When he finished, I was in severe pain everywhere and wet from sweating as if I had just stepped out of a swimming pool. He said the word *fibromyalgia*, but I was too out of it at the time to respond even with a question mark. I sat and cried with pain as he left the room.

When he came back, he had written down the names of a couple of Web sites, saying that some doctors think fibromyalgia is a myth, or that it is actually myofacial pain syndrome with a twist, or that it's all in the head. That's because there is no proof that it exists—medically, that is.

Great. I had a nonexistent *syndrome* with a weird name.

"So how do you fix it?" I asked.

He shook his head and wrote me two prescriptions for Elavil and Flexeril.

I was starting to feel a bit better with the help of the prescriptions. At least I was sleeping better. Then about six weeks later, I woke up one morning and my neck hurt so badly I couldn't turn my head. Dr. Bhatt gave me trigger point injections in the back of my neck and shoulder area. In a few days I was to start doing some gentle neck and shoulder exercises as a follow-up to these injections so that those muscles wouldn't freeze up again. I still do them—and more.

But several days after that flare, a number of the other symptoms began to ease back into my life. I could see the writing on the wall. Raise the dosage, then a month or so later raise it again, then again. This was a merry-go-round I was not willing to stay on. I didn't want to keep raising the dose and become dependant on these for the rest of my life. So I asked him if there was something natural I could use.

Dr. Bhatt recommended two supplements, which I bought that day at Walmart. Then I forged ahead and began my research in depth. The bits and pieces I was assembling confirmed what he had said. Many doctors did not believe in fibromyalgia. That alone was unbelievable! *Look at me and the shape I'm in*, I thought. But now I was on the road to feeling better!

I thank God every day that this relatively young doctor knew his stuff. Back in 1998, fibromyalgia was not a common syndrome, much less a common word. Dr. Bhatt had given me *hope*. He enabled me to raise the quality of my life—he literally gave me back my life.

Throughout the course of these years with fibromyalgia, my life has changed dramatically. I had given up my dream job of nine years with the Department of Natural Resources. But then, even with fibromyalgia, I got *and kept* a job working part time at a large retail store for the next nine years. I am retired now and writing. I am hosting a very successful fibromyalgia support group, full of wonderful people where we all learn, share, support, and help one another. I attend book signing events and local expos and stay productive.

I still have fibromyalgia. After all, it is a chronic condition and doesn't go away. But I have learned to manage my symptoms quite successfully by eating appropriately, using stress management techniques, moving, taking the appropriate supplements *for me*, pacing myself, and avoiding the things that aggravate my symptoms. I've learned how to side-step flare-ups. And if I do get one, about six per year now, I can look back and see exactly what I did to create it. And the next time I can avoid it altogether.

I still pace myself and do deep breathing exercises daily. I do tai chi and meditate every day too. I eat appropriately and take my supplements. And there are lots of little things I do, as I describe in the following section. And I will continue to do all of these things. All in all, it's a wonderful new lifestyle ... that works for me!

Adapting to Fibromyalgia

For one year I was unable to hold a job. I used this time to research and to find the right balance of things to do for me and my symptoms to bring my body back to a semblance of normal. (Fortunately, you have in your hands the benefit of that research, and it won't take you nearly as long!) Then I began working part time at a large retail store. I learned that I had to change my shoes three times a day because what was comfortable in the morning was no longer comfortable at noon. Even though each pair was a good supportive shoe, I wore a half size larger shoe in the afternoon when my feet hurt and swelled. Then I changed into a different style of shoe when I got home.

In the beginning I couldn't sit in my then new La-Z-Boy, so I got a secondhand Bentwood rocker, which is now "my chair." I couldn't sit in my car for more than ten minutes without experiencing severe pain, so I had my car seat reupholstered—the seat was filled in with foam so that it was level, and the lumbar pad was removed. I wear sunglasses year round. I have two pairs in the car and always have a pair in my purse. I keep a pair of sunglasses next to my computer for those times when the computer screen seems too bright. The new HD sunglasses actually work quite well.

I never used to take pills—not even aspirin. Now I take up to seven supplements three times a day. I was never a breakfast person, but I did learn to eat in the morning because I need the energy and my supplements are best taken with food. I no longer drink carbonated drinks. I eat a lot more whole fresh foods than I ever did before and much less sugar and fewer sweets. (I really learned to love fresh veggies—who would have guessed?)

I bought a rubber cone-shaped gizmo so I could open jars and milk containers because I have no grip in my hands. I have scissors in every room to open everything from a bag of cereal to a new CD to a new box of antihistamines to a new package of roller ball pens. I buy the large bodied pens so I can hold them more easily.

I used to drink coffee by the potful. Now I drink only two cups of coffee a day, and they are both half hot water and half coffee. I drink lots of water and green tea. I put one packet of Just Like Sugar in my green tea. With a pH of eight, it helps to keep my body's pH on the alkaline side, just as the fruits and veggies do. Before fibromyalgia, this would never have occurred to me. But I've learned that chronic illness *thrives* in an acidic environment. So I try to be conscious of maintaining a more alkaline diet. The Juice Plus+ I take helps this cause, and it also has nearly all the antioxidants I need each day.

I ask the grocery bagger to fill my canvas bags lightly, and I make more trips bringing them into the house—more exercise. I keep everything in its proper place so when fibro-fog hits I can still find it. Almost. I always keep gloves handy so I can hold a cold glass of water or take frozen food out of the freezer. In a restaurant, I wrap a napkin around my glass of ice water so my hands don't hurt while holding it.

I do the dishes in two stages, sitting to rest periodically. I change the bed sheets, vacuum, clean the bathroom, and do laundry the same way, of course.

I bought a sleep number bed (I am a number forty). My pillow is one-third of a feather pillow—a full size pillow forces my chin down and blocks my airway—so I cut the feather pillow into three pieces. (That was fun!) I do toe and ankle exercises before I get out of bed. I do neck and shoulder exercises often during the day. I meditate and do tai chi exercises every morning and sometimes in the afternoon.

I very rarely go out after nine p.m. I use the hour before my ten o'clock bedtime to wind down and relax. I don't attend large public events where the noise would be intolerable. I always have earplugs in my purse anyway. I never know when I will go to a movie with the grandkids. And, of course, I have a long-sleeved flannel or fleece shirt in the car in case it's cold in the movie theater. I learned early on that planning ahead is always a good idea.

Another thing I always carry in my purse is box of mints. It's my first-aid kit to nausea and flatulence. Peppermint oil (not simply mint-flavor but the oil) is a must to have on hand. Thank you, Junior Mints.

I bought a painter's facemask to cover my nose and mouth when my husband is painting or working in the basement with paint thinners and such or when I use bleach or Comet to clean the tub or sinks.

I always have that fleece jacket or fleece wrap nearby even in the summer, to keep air-conditioning drafts and chills off my neck, shoulders, hips, and knees. I bought several "fleece pieces"—remnants from the fabric store for $1.50. I wrap my knees or shoulders or upper arms in them as I watch TV or read.

I bought a winter coat that zips up over my chin and has a hood to keep the wind chill off the tender points. I buy only loose-fitting comfortable clothing. I learned quickly about the negative effects of tight jeans and turtlenecks.

I try to stay upbeat. Fortunately, I still have my sense of humor. I wear light colored clothes. I watch uplifting or funny movies. I listen to soothing or light tempo music. I play with my cats. I read lighthearted, romantic, mystery novels. I surround myself with light-colored walls, brightly colored accents, and the things I enjoy. I have learned to lift my life.

These are a few of my life adaptations to fibromyalgia. But I am now able to sit at my computer, while exercising my feet and ankles regularly, long enough to research and write this book. Fibromyalgia is still with me. But by using a few little tricks described here—supplements, meditation, deep breathing exercises, tai chi exercises, and avoiding my aggravators— I have been able to manage my fibromyalgia. I still have a bad day now and then, but doesn't everyone? I haven't had the need to visit my doctor for fibromyalgia symptoms since the year 2000!

If I can help other souls learn to manage their fibromyalgia symptoms by recognizing their aggravators, learning to pace their activities, and become more conscious of foods that can aggravate symptoms, then I consider my mission accomplished.

Everyone is different, and what works for one may not work for everyone. But the more you know, the better you are able to choose wisely. It is my desire to show you more options to ease your pain. I thank God for the opportunity and the wherewithal to do so.

Endnotes

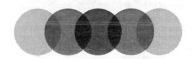

Chapter 1

1. WebMD.com. What is Fibromyalgia? Are Women More Likely to Get Fibromyalgia Than Men? http://www.webmd.com/fibromyalgia/guide/arthritis-fibromyalgia. Accessed May 15, 2010.

2. National Institute of Arthritis and Musculoskeletal and Skin Diseases (NIAMS), Health Information, Fibromyalgia, Questions and Answers About Fibromyalgia http://www.

niams.nih.gov/Health_Info/Fibromyalgia/
default.asp Accessed May 15, 2010.

3. Starlanyl, Devin and Copeland, Mary Ellen. *Fibromyalgia and Chronic Myofacial Pain Syndrome, Second Edition.* 2001. CA, New Harbringer Publications, Inc. p125.

4. University of Maryland Medical Center (UMM). Medical Reference. Encyclopedia Fibromyalgia, Symptoms http://www.umm.edu/ency/article/000427sym.htm. Accessed May 15, 2010.

5. WebMd.com. Fibromyalgia Guide, Overview and Facts, Fibromyalgia and sleep. Why Can't I Sleep at Night With Fibromyalgia? http://www.webmd.com/fibromyalgia/guide/fibro-mayalgia-and-sleep Accessed May 15, 2010.

6. University of Michigan Health System (UMHS). Fibromyalgia. Self-Management Skills and Techniques- Sleep. Williams, D.A. and Carey, M. You Really Need To Sleep. Why is sleep so essential? 2003. PDF/Adobe Acrobat. Available

at: http://www.med.umich.edu/painresearch/patients/sleep.pdf Accessed May 15, 2010.

7. UMHS. Chronic Pain and Research Center- for Patients. Fibromyalgia- Diagnosis. 1996. Available at: http://www.med.umich.edu/painresearch/pro/diagnosis.htm Accessed May 15, 2010.

8. Ibid.

9. Fibromyalgia and Fatigue Centers, Inc. Fibromyalgia. http://www.fibroandfatigue.com/fibromyalgia.html Accessed May 15, 2010.

10. University of Maryland Medical Center (UMM). Medical reference-Encyclopedia. Fibromyalgia Overview, Causes, incidence and risk factors. 2009. Available at: http://www.umm.edu/ency/article/000427.htm Accessed may 15, 2010.

11. WebMD. Fibromyalgia Guide, Overview and Facts, Fibromyalgia Causes. http://www.webmd.com/fibromyalgia/guide/fibromyalgia-causes Accessed May 15, 2010.

12. WebMD. Fibromyalgia Guide, Overview and Facts, Fibromyalgia Causes, Other Theories About Causes of Fibromyalgia. http://www.webmd.com/fibromyalgia/guide/fibromyalgia-causes Accessed May 15, 2010.

13. Womentowomen.com, Search: Fibromyalgia. Treating fibromyalgia naturally–so you can shine again, Stress, hormonal balance and fibro-myalgia–what's the connection? http://www.womentowomen.com/fatigueandstress/fibro-myalgia.aspx Accessed May 15, 2010.

14. University of Maryland Medical Center (UMM). Medical reference-Encyclopedia. Fibromyalgia Overview, Causes, incidence and risk factors. 2009. Available at: http://www.umm.edu/ency/article/000427.htm Accessed May 15, 2010.

Chapter 2

15. UMM.edu, Fibromyalgia, Symptoms, Signs and Tests http://www.umm.edu/ency/article/000427sym.htm. Accessed May 15, 2010.

16. UMHS. Chronic Pain and Research- For Patients. Fibromyalgia-Diagnosis. 1996. Available at: http://www.med.umich.edu/painresearch/pro/fibromyalgia.htm Accessed May 15, 2010.

17. UMM. Altmed, Condition, Fibromyalgia. Introduction. http://www.umm.edu/altmed/articles/fibromyalgia-000061.htm. Accessed May 15, 2010.

18. UMHS. Department of Public Relations, Newsroom, Nov 28, 2006. "The pain from fibromyalgia is real, researchers say." http://www.med.umich.edu/opm/newspage/2006/fibromyalgia.htm. Accessed May 15, 2010.

19. WebMD. Fibromyalgia Guide, Fibromyalgia Treatment and Care, p2. http://www.webmd.com/fibromyalgia/guide/fibromyalgia-treatments?page=2 Accessed May 15, 2010.

20. UMM.Altmed-Articles-S-adenosylmethionine. Fibromyalgia. http://www.umm.edu/altmed/articles/s-adenosylmethionine-000324.htm. Accessed May 15, 2010.

21. WebMD. Fibromyalgia Guide, Home Remedies, Fibromyalgia and exercise. http://www.webmd.com/fibromyalgia/guide/fibromyalgia-and-exercise Accessed May 15, 2010. .

22. MedicineNet.com. Chronic Pain Center, A-Z, Pain Management: Trigger Point Injections (TPI). http://www.medicinenet.com/trigger_point_injection/article.htm Accessed May 15, 2010.

23. WebMD. Fibromyalgia Guide, Fibromyalgia Treatment and Care, p2. http://www.webmd.com/fibromyalgia/guide/fibromyalgia-treatments?page=2 Accessed May 15, 2010.

Chapter 3

24. National Fibromyalgia Partnership. Fibromyalgia Overview, Other conditions Associated with FM, Stiffness http://www.fmpartnership.org/Files/Website2005/Learn%20About%20Fibromyalgia/FM%20overview/Monograph—English.htm Accessed May 15, 2010.

25. Oelke, J. *Natural Choices for Fibromyalgia*. 2001. MI: Natural Choices, Inc. pp 35–36.

26. UMHS. Fibromyalgia. "Improve Your Functioning Through Effective Pacing" Williams, D.A. and Carey, M. 2003. PDF/Adobe Acrobat. http://www.med.umich.edu/painresearch/patients/pacing.pdf Accessed May 15, 2010.

27. Ibid.

28. Womentowomen.com, Search: Fibromyalgia. Treating fibromyalgia naturally–so you can shine again, Stress, hormonal balance and fibromyalgia–what's the connection? Adrenal glands. http://www.womentowomen.com/fatigueand-stress/fibromyalgia.aspx Accessed May 15, 2010.

29. Teitelbaum, Jacob, M.D. *From Fatigued to Fantastic*. 2007. New York, Penguin Group, p 25.

30. UMHS. Health Topics A-Z. Fibromyalgia. How is it treated? 2007. Available at: http://www.med.umich.edu/11ibr/aha/umfibromyalgia.htm Accessed May 15, 2010.

31. NFA. An Overview for the Newly Diagnosed Patient. Treatment of Fibromyalgia. http://www.fmaware.org/site/PageServer?pagename=fibromyalgia_overview Accessed May 15, 2010.

32. Ibid.

Chapter 4

33. WebMD. Fibromyalgia Guide, Home Remedies, Fibromyalgia: The Diet Connection, Seven Foods To Avoid. http://www.webmd.com/fibromyalgia/guide/fibromyalgia-the-diet-connection Accessed May 15, 2010.

34. Colbert, Don, M.D., *Seven Pillars of Health*, 2007. Siloam. p 82.

35. www.rheumatic.org/sugar.htm Accessed May 15, 2010.

36. Drugs.com. Natural Products. "L." L-Theanine. http://www.drugs.com/npc/1-theanine.html Accessed May 15, 2010.

37. Oelke, J, N.D., Ph.D. *Natural Choices for Fibromyalgia*. 2001. MI: Natural Choices, Inc. pp 129–131.

38. Women To Women. Explore our Knowledge, Digestion and GI Health, Gluten Intolerance. http://www.womentowomen.com/digestion-andgihealth/glutenintolerance.aspx Accessed May 15, 2010.

39. National Digestive Diseases Information Clearinghouse. Div of NIH. A-Z List of Digestive Diseases, Lactose Intolerance. http://digestive.niddk.nih.gov/ddiseases/pubs/lacto-seintolerance/ Accessed May 15, 2010.

40. Teitelbaum, Jacob, M.D. *From Fatigued to Fantastic*. 2007. New York, Penguin Group, p 119–122.

41. UMM. Medical Reference-Complimentary Medicine-Omega 3. 2007. Available at: http://www.umm.edu/altmed/articles/omega-3-000316.htm Accessed May 15, 2010.

42. NIH. Office of Dietary Supplements. Omega 3 Fatty Acids and Health. 2005. Available at: http://www.ods.od.nih.gov/FactSheets/Omega3FattyAcidsandHealth_pf.asp Accessed May 15, 2010.

43. University of Cincinnati, Ohio State University. Health Topics, Complimentary Medicine, Omega-3, "Understanding Omega-3 and Omega-6." http://www.netwellness.org/healthtopics/alternative/Omega3.cfm Accessed May 15, 2010.

44. NIH. National Center for Biotechnology. Pubmed, Omega 3. The Center for Genetics, Nutrition and Health, Washington, D.C. http://www.ncbi.nlm.nih.gov/pubmed/12442909 .Accessed May 15, 2010.

45. FDA. Food, Food Safety, Product Specific Information, "What You Need To Know About Mercury in Fish And Shellfish." http://www.fda.gov/Food/FoodSafety/Product-SpecificInformation/Seafood/FoodbornePathogensContaminants/

Methylmercury/ucm115662.htm Accessed May 15, 2010.

46. Oelke, J. Natural Choices for Fibromyalgia. 2001. MI: Natural Choices, Inc. pp107–110.

47. UMM. Medical Reference-Complimentary Medicine-Omega 3. 2007. Available at: http://www.umm.edu/altmed/articles/omega-3-000316.htm Accessed May 15, 2010.

Chapter 5

48. Fibromyalgia-Symptoms.org, Medical Treatment, Frequency Microcurrent. http://www.fibromy-algia-symptoms.org/fibromyalgia_fsm.html Accessed May 15, 2010.

49. Nexalin Therapy. http://nexalintherapy.com/ Accessed May 15, 2010.

Chapter 6

50. Teitelbaum, Jacob, M.D. *From Fatigued to Fantastic.* 2007. New York, Penguin Group, p 218.

51. Ibid

52. Pubmed.com, Treatment of Fibromyalgia Syndrome with Super Malic Acid: a randomized, double-blind placebo-controlled, crossover pilot study by Russell, Michalek, Flechas, and Abraham, 1995. http://www.ncbi.nlm.nih.gov/pubmed/8587088?itool=EntrezSystem2.PEntrez.Pubmed.Pubmed_ResultsPanel.Pubmed_RVDocSumandordinalpos=2 Accessed May 15, 2010.

53. Healing With Nutrition, Fibromyalgia, Missing Nutrients linked to Fibromyalgia and Chronic Pain. http://www.healingwithnutrition.com/fdisease/fibromyalgia/magnesiumstudy.html Accessed May15, 2010.

54. UMM. Medical Reference, Complementary Medicine, Supplements, Alpha Lipoic Acid. http://www.umm.edu/altmed/articles/alpha-lipoic-000285.htm Accessed May 15, 2010.

55. MedlinePlus.gov. Site search, "Antioxidants," Antioxidants. www.nlm.nih.gov/medlineplus/antioxidants.html. Accessed May 15, 2010.

56. WomentoWomen.com. Site Search, "Vitamin D," "Is Vitamin D deficiency casting a cloud over your health?" http://www.womento-women.com/healthynutrition/vitamind.aspx Accessed May 15, 2010.

57. UMM. Medical Reference, Complementary Medicine, Supplements, CoenzymeQ10, How To Take It. http://www.umm.edu/altmed/articles/coenzyme-q10–000295.htm Accessed May 15, 2010.

58. UMM. Medical Reference, Complimentary Medicine, Herb, Siberian Ginseng, How To Take It. http://www.umm.edu/altmed/articles/siberian-ginseng-000250.htm Accessed May 15, 2010.

59. Drugs.com. Site Search, "Rhodiola," Rhodiola: Natural Product Monograph. http://www.drugs.com/npp/rhodiola.html Accessed May 15, 2010.

60. UMM. Medical Reference, Complimentary Medicine, Supplements, S-adenosylmethionine, How To Take It. http://www.umm.edu/altmed/articles/s-adenosylmethionine-000324.htm Accessed May 15, 2010.

61. UMM. Medical Reference , Complementary Medicine, Herb, Garlic. http://www.umm.edu/altmed/articles/garlic-000245.htm Accessed May 15, 2010.

62. Pubmed.gov. Site search, "Olive Leaf Extract," "Assessment of Anti-inflammatory and Antinociceptive properties of Olea europaea L. 2010. Journal of Medicinal Food. http://www.ncbi.nlm.nih.gov/pubmed/20132039?itool=EntrezSystem2.PEntrez.Pubmed.Pubmed_ResultsPanel.Pubmed_RVDocSumandordinalpos=1 Accessed May 15, 2010.

63. TheWolfeClinic.com. Site Search, "Oil of oregano," Super Strength Oil Of Oregano. http://www.thewolfeclinic.com/oregano.html Accessed May 15, 2010.

64. UMM. Medical Reference , Complementary Medicine, Supplement, 5-HTP. http://www.umm.edu/altmed/articles/5-hydroxytrypto-phan-000283.htm Accessed May 15, 2010.

65. UMM. Medical Reference, Complementary Medicine, Supplement, Melatonin. http://www.umm.edu/altmed/articles/melatonin-000315.htm Accessed May 15, 2010.

66. Teitelbaum, Jacob, M.D. *From Fatigued to Fantastic*. 2007. New York, Penguin Group, p 59.

67. American Journal of Clinical Nutrition. www.ajcn.org, search result for June 1, 2009 issue, "Multivitamin use and telomere length in women." Abstract. http://www.ajcn.org/cgi/search?sortspec=relevanc eandauthor1=andfulltext=Multivitamin%2C+DN Aandpubdate_year=2009andvolume=andfirstpage Accessed May 15, 2010.

68. Colbert, Don, M.D. *The Seven Pillars of Health*. Siloam 2007. p 5

69. Oelke, J, N.D., Ph.D. *Natural Choices for Fibromyalgia*. 2001. MI: Natural Choices, Inc. pp 123–128.

Chapter 7

70. UMHS. Fibromyalgia. Self-Management Skills and Techniques-Pleasant Activities. Williams, D.A. and Carey, M. You Really Need To Sleep. 2003. PDF/Adobe Acrobat. Available at: http://www.med.umich.edu/painresearch/patients/sleep.pdf Accessed May 15, 2010.

Index

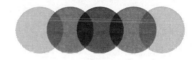

for more information or
to contact the author, please visit:

ManagingFibromyalgia.com
PatiChandlerJuicePlus.com

or

facebook.com/FibromyalgiaNaturallywithPatiChandler

listen|imagine|view|experience

AUDIO BOOK DOWNLOAD INCLUDED WITH THIS BOOK!

In your hands you hold a complete digital entertainment package. Besides purchasing the paper version of this book, this book includes a free download of the audio version of this book. Simply use the code listed below when visiting our website. Once downloaded to your computer, you can listen to the book through your computer's speakers, burn it to an audio CD or save the file to your portable music device (such as Apple's popular iPod) and listen on the go!

How to get your free audio book digital download:

1. Visit www.tatepublishing.com and click on the e|LIVE logo on the home page.
2. Enter the following coupon code:
   8a9d-94cf-0ec1-b1b7-74b7-5354-afbd-c63d
3. Download the audio book from your e|LIVE digital locker and begin enjoying your new digital entertainment package today!